Oxford Medical Publications

The End of Adolescence

The End of Adolescence

Philip Graham

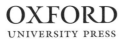
OXFORD
UNIVERSITY PRESS

OXFORD

UNIVERSITY PRESS

Great Clarendon Street, Oxford OX2 6DP

Oxford University Press is a department of the University of Oxford.
It furthers the University's objective of excellence in research, scholarship,
and education by publishing worldwide in

Oxford   New York

Auckland   Bangkok   Buenos Aires   Cape Town   Chennai
Dar es Salaam   Delhi   Hong Kong   Istanbul   Karachi   Kolkata
Kuala Lumpur   Madrid   Melbourne   Mexico City   Mumbai   Nairobi
São Paulo   Shanghai   Taipei   Tokyo   Toronto

Oxford is a registered trade mark of Oxford University Press
in the UK and in certain other countries

Published in the United States
by Oxford University Press Inc., New York

A catalogue record for this title is available from the British Library
Library of Congress Cataloging in Publication Data

(Data available)

ISBN 0 19 8526245 (Pbk)

10 9 8 7 6 5 4 3 2 1

Typeset by Cepha Imaging Pvt. Ltd, Bangalore, India
Printed in Great Britain
on acid-free paper by Biddles Ltd, King's Lynn

Acknowledgements

I have had useful discussions about different aspects of this book's contents with the following, all of whom have been generous with their encouragement: Jill Barton, Michael Burawoy, George and Moira Cyriax, Paul Ennals, Nori Graham, Anna Graham, Daniel Graham, David Graham, Peter Hindmarsh, Robin and Inge Hyman, Bryan Lask, John and Janet Murphy, Stanley and Judy Price, Laurence and Mary Shurman, Gillian Tindall, Barbara Tizard, Dan Weisselberg and Susan Woollacott.

I am especially grateful to Nicola Hilliard, Lisa Payne, and Marjorie Smith who read and made comments on the whole of the book in its penultimate draft.

The publications of the Trust for the Study of Adolescence, founded and led by John Coleman, have been an invaluable source of information. The members of the staff of the Library and Information Centre of the National Children's Bureau, London have gone out of their way to be helpful throughout.

It has taken me a long time to write this book and I have had many helpful discussions about the ideas in it with friends and colleagues. I apologise to those whom I have failed to list, though I suspect some may be grateful not to be associated with some of the more provocative suggestions I have made. Of course, those I have listed should in no way be regarded as endorsing any of the book's contents.

CONTENTS

Introduction

Now that women have been liberated, the grey power of the elderly has been asserted, racism is publicly ostracized, and facilities for the disabled are legally required in all public places, the teens have become the last group whose disempowerment is invisible because it is so much taken for granted. In many ways, of course, the teens are only too visible—they are always making the headlines. But too often these merely confirm their stigmatized position in society. The word 'adolescent' has again become, as it has in the past, a term of condescending mockery.

In this book I have tried to take a critical look at the way western society thinks about and treats those in their teen years. I have then gone on to suggest ways in which the adult world might rethink its attitudes to the young so that they are more in line with the way they think and behave rather than with the way those in the media and even sometimes those who write textbooks make them out to be.

In the first chapter, I have tried to give an idea of the diversity of teenage life and personality, suggesting that such diversity defeats all attempts at generalizations about the teen years. I then go on to describe some of the myths about adolescence and the travesty of the truth they represent. I suggest that the idea that the teen years are a separate phase of life, clearly different from the years that come before and after is seriously flawed. I introduce one of the main themes of the book—the ways in which adult society fails to take into account the competence of young people and refuses to allow them to use their skills. The adult world, I suggest, infantilizes and disempowers young people, often with disastrous consequences. In Chapter 2, I provide a historical account of the development of modern day views about adolescence. I suggest that the evidence from historical times and from studies of traditional societies, even from non-human primates, strongly suggests that adolescence is what the adult world makes of it rather than that there is any particularly 'natural' way for the young to behave.

In Chapter 3, I discuss the different ways in which parents and those in their teens interact together and how the evidence strongly suggests that the best outcomes for children's personalities occur when parents begin by carefully observing the way their children feel and behave in different circumstances when they are infants and toddlers, responding to them as individuals. If they then go on to consult them and respect their views in the primary school years, and move to sharing decision-making with them when they reach their teens, the chances that their children will enter adulthood in good mental health are further increased. In Chapter 4, I begin by pointing to the fact that most teenagers are no more moody or miserable than the rest of us and then look at some of the myths surrounding depression and suicide in the teens. I go on to suggest that when the young are miserable and unhappy, it is the powerless predicament in which they find themselves that is often responsible. Lacking control over events affecting them is a depressing experience for people of all ages. What makes adolescence different is the way the whole age group is disempowered.

Most young people in their teens do not get involved in antisocial behaviour but, given the way they are sometimes treated, are amazingly compliant and obedient. In Chapter 5, I discuss the ways in which, when antisocial behaviour arises for the first time in the teen years, for a substantial proportion of those young people involved, though certainly not for that substantial minority who have been seriously disruptive since their early years, the powerless social situation of the young is partly responsible. In this chapter, I introduce the notion that if we treated those in their teens more as young adults and those who had not reached this age much more as children requiring more protection than we currently give them, we might do better by them. The notion of adolescence as an in-between age that is neither one thing nor the other seems to result in our failing to protect young children as well as infantilization of the competent teens. This leads naturally to the conclusion that the age of criminal responsibility should be raised from 10 years to 14 years.

In Chapter 6, dealing with sexual behaviour, I look first at the myth of sexual promiscuity among teenagers. I then go on to discuss the way in which the adult world disempowers those in this age group as far as their sexual behaviour is concerned, failing to provide them with adequate information or with the wherewithal to practice safe sex. Many teenagers want to behave responsibly, but the rules do not permit their competence to be recognized. I suggest that if the age of consent in girls were reduced from 16 to the more realistic age of 14 years, as it is in many countries with a better record of teenage conceptions, this would not result in an increase in sexual behaviour, but would enable those who do engage in it to behave more safely.

Chapter 7 discusses the use of alcohol and drugs in the young. Here I point out that the main influence on the consumption is the amount the adult population consumes. I suggest that if the emphasis were changed from stopping those in their teens from drinking alcohol to strong discouragement of binge drinking and heavier penalties for alcohol-fuelled physical aggression at all ages, the young would almost certainly drink less. I suggest that the law relating to entry of those in their teens into pubs and to purchases from off-licenses should be reviewed with a view to bringing it more into line with the real world. The young are also, I suggest, especially sensitive to the hypocrisy involved in health warnings about the so-called 'soft' drugs. In the next chapter, I discuss how, as the young enter their teens too many of them are already literally burdened with overweight arising from unhealthy food and too little exercise. How can the adult world criticize the young for their tendency either to overeat or to diet to the point of anorexia if it has allowed a situation to develop in which so many young people enter their teens in such an unhealthy state?

In Chapter 9, I celebrate the success of that majority of secondary schools in which those in their teens make remarkable academic progress, taught as they are, by dedicated staff. But there is sound evidence that school is an unpopular and unrewarding experience for many young people. I suggest that, while the diversity of educational need makes it difficult to provide for the requirements of all students, it would be highly desirable if ways forward included a more life-relevant curriculum, considerably more opportunity for teacher–student interaction than is the case at present, and a greater degree of student participation in the running of schools.

Those in their teens spend more of their waking time out of school than in it. In Chapter 10, I discuss how the replacement of productive work in the life of the teens by a massive amount of leisure time has not been accompanied by any equivalent effort to provide rewarding ways in which such 'free' time might be spent. Similarly, the rules and regulations regarding the amount those in their teens are allowed to work reflects once again attitudes in adult society that infantilize inexperienced but highly competent young people.

Finally, in the last chapter, I discuss ways in which the competence of young people might be acknowledged and used productively in the neighbourhoods in which they live. Children, or pre-teens, would, I suggest, have a better deal if they were much better protected and prepared for a future in the 'real' world than they are at present. In contrast, once they reach their teens, we should stop infantilizing young people and allow them to reclaim the independence to which their competence entitles them. Bringing the voting age down from 18 to 16 and then, having judged the effect of this change, maybe even to 14 years, would be a powerful signal that the adult world recognized the level of competence and understanding of young people. It might also mark the beginning of the end for the largely unhelpful concept of adolescence so widespread in western society today.

I have written this book for the general public, especially those who are interested in taking a fresh look at the 'youth problem'. Although I have occasionally made suggestions to parents about the way they might respond to their teenage children, this is not intended to be a 'How to do it' book for such parents. I feel poorly qualified to instruct parents and the young how to behave. In any case, there are some excellent, recently published 'How to do it' guides for parents of middle class teenagers. I have listed some at the end of the book. All the same, I think the book will be of particular interest to parents of children just about to be or already in their teens, secondary school teachers, and to that large number of those in their teens who, given half a chance, are really interested in issues involving them and affecting their lives.

This is also not a textbook. It is not a comprehensive account of adolescent life. For example, there are no separate chapters on issues central to adolescent life such as friendships or teenage culture, because these subjects are not relevant to my disempowerment theme. Nor have I provided weighty details of all the books and journal articles backing up each statement, though all the statements I have made are well backed by evidence, apart from some key references listed at the end of the book. I hope though that tutors in child development, sociology, and psychology who think their students might respond to a provocative text, will find it useful. There are some excellent, non-controversial, recently published textbooks, especially on the psychology of adolescence. Again, I have listed a couple of these at the end of the book.

This book is written from three different standpoints. On the one hand, I have tried to use a long clinical experience as a child and adolescent psychiatrist seeing individual young people with problems. If one only sees people with problems, however, one comes away with a distorted view of the world. I have therefore also used quite extensive experience gained by interviewing so-called 'normal' children, young people, and their parents in population studies, as well as in supervising research of this nature. Finally, my involvement in voluntary organizations concerned with social, educational, and health policy development, means I have been engaged over many years in debating desirable policy changes affecting young people. In my working life, I have felt that each of these types of experience has enriched the others. Whether this book has gained in a similar way, I shall have to leave it to the reader to judge.

Chapter 1

The unpopular age

1.1 Please don't let me be an adolescent!

In Edward Albee's play 'Finding the Sun', a boy, Fergus, reflects on his age. He tells a 70-year-old man, Henden, that he is 16 years old. Henden responds 'Don't be silly'. 'A lot of people say that', replies Fergus. Henden says, 'There is no such age'.

Later, Fergus is talking to Abigail, a young woman seven years older than he is. She tells him he's an adolescent. Fergus explodes 'Adolescent. If there's one thing an adolescent doesn't want to be called it's an adolescent—even those of us *know* we're adolescents, accept it, we don't want the word used: we don't like the sound of it. Ad-o-les-cent; it's an ugly word'. Abigail asks 'What would you like to be called?' Fergus suggests 'Young man?' Abigail considers 'Young man. That has a nice sound. *You* are a … young man'.

As a psychiatrist working for over 25 years in a children's hospital, I have listened and talked to young men and women of Fergus's age referred for emotional and behavioural problems. As a researcher over an even longer period of time, I have been involved in studies of 'ordinary' school students of this age who were selected at random from school populations and from 'young people' on lists of family doctors. Some of these lived in very deprived areas, others were much better off. As a university teacher, I have discussed issues to do with adolescence with undergraduates, themselves only just out of their teenage years. Finally, like everyone else, I have learned about the teenage years from my own adolescence, as well as that of members of my family and friends.

1.2 The typical 'teenager'? Forget it!

Over many years I have often asked those in their teens what their lives are like at the present time. Here are some examples of the sorts of answers I have been given. The replies that follow are imaginary, but they are drawn from real accounts given to me by teenagers I have encountered in a number of different ways over the years.

Fourteen-year-old James: 'What is my life like at the moment? Well, to be honest, it's not all that good. It's very confusing. I always thought Mum and

Dad were getting on pretty well together, and just a few weeks ago, Mum sat me and June down and said Dad was leaving. He was going to live with someone else. Or he thought he was. He was going to live by himself for a few months and then decide whether he wanted to live with this other person or not. Or he might want to live by himself, but he definitely didn't want to live with us. It seems he and Mum have been talking or rather arguing about this for months, and we never knew. Well, it's not quite true to say we never knew. Because I did hear them arguing once when they didn't know I was listening. But I had sort of forgotten about it. It was a real shock. So now Dad has gone, and I go and see him in his room a couple of times a week. But I don't know if I should go. Mum doesn't seem very pleased about it. She seems more pleased with June. She won't even talk to him on the phone. She just won't go and see him, even though he keeps on asking her to. I spend as much time as I can with Mum, because she cries a lot of the time. I keep on telling her to cheer up. She'll find someone else. He isn't worth it. But that just seems to make her angry. I've got no one to ask what to say to her. I can't talk to friends at school. I'd feel too embarrassed to do that. Sort of letting my Mum down'.

Sixteen-year-old Janet: 'What is my life like at the moment? I think I have a great life, to be honest. School's a bit of a laugh. I don't take it all that seriously, but I get by. I don't s'pose I'll do that well in my GCSEs, but too bad. There's other things in life. I have a great time at the weekend. Saturday I do checkout at Sainsbury's and earn a bit. Then in the evening I spend a bit or rather more than a bit, I reckon. Me and Babs, my friend, go for a drink at a pub we know where they're not too fussy about your age, and then we go clubbing. Take a couple of 'E's and have a really great time till about two. Go mad really. Then we usually pick up a couple of blokes and take them to Bab's sister's place. She doesn't mind what we do. She has a rotten life with her little baby crying all the time. She reckons we ought to have a good time while we can, and she's got this extra room that just got mattresses in it. So we have a lot of fun and then in the morning we kick them out and have a laugh and then we go back to sleep and then we get up around two and then we don't do nothing much, except watch a video till we go back home and go to bed. Mum usually has a go at me, but she can't talk much. Look at the life she leads. More dope than us, you bet. And miserable with it'.

Seventeen-year-old Mark: 'What sort of a life do I have at the moment? Well, you might not call it much of a life, but I get by OK. Felt great last weekend. A dozen beers and half a grain of Charlie up my nose. Monday not so great then Tuesday, yesterday, got real low again and needed more stuff. Nicked a couple of mobile phones off blokes who was using them, one at Euston and the other some little geezer on the top of a bus when I got away from there.

Real startled they looked. Sold 'em off for just enough for another good snort so I'm OK now'.

Eighteen-year-old Yasmin: 'What sort of a life do I have at the moment? Pretty good, I think. I suppose I'm pretty work-focused, and you might think that's wrong. I've just got the result of my A's and I've just done well enough to go to the University that's my first choice. I don't think I have a very exciting life, but that's OK by me. As well as school work, and now I'm trying to read the stuff the University has sent me that I need to know before I start my course, I do quite a bit of sport. I work out twice a week at a gym and play tennis with my Mum and Dad on Sundays. I do look after myself and try not to put on weight. My Mum gets on at me if she sees me stuffing myself, and I'm grateful to her for that, though I do think I know myself what I can eat and what I can't. I have two good girlfriends, a bit like me. I don't have a boyfriend, never have, not serious, though a lot of boys have tried to get off with me. Well, maybe just one or two. I think I have a reputation for being a bit untouchable. But I think I'm going to keep that stuff till I go to University and even then I'm not sure. I think I'm going to wait until I meet someone I really like and then go for it'.

Fifteen-year-old Jennifer: 'What's my life like at the moment? I don't know why, but it seems pretty terrible. I don't know what's wrong with me. I just don't know how to shake this mood off. I feel awful. I ought to feel really lucky. I've got my Mum and Dad at home, and loads of my friends have separated parents. We're not poor. We're definitely not poor. I get everything I ask for, really. But I just feel there's this great black cloud. I did take about twenty of my Mum's depression tablets about a month ago, and had to go to Casualty for a washout. They just sent me home and told me not to be a silly girl and not to do it again. My Dad says it's ridiculous a girl my age thinking I'm depressed. Girls my age don't get depressed. I have thought of going to the doctor, but I'm pretty sure he would say the same as my Dad. I just don't know what it's all due to. I know the family dog died a year ago, but I wasn't that fond of her anyway. Then one of my two friends wouldn't have anything more to do with me a couple of months ago. She said I was boring. Well, I expect I am. I just don't know what to do about it'.

Sixteen-year-old Amisha: 'What's my life like at the moment? What do you think? It was just about alright until three weeks ago. Up to then I had rows with my Dad about music and friends and stuff, but school was good. I was doing pretty well and with my friends, we used to have a laugh. I really looked forward to Mondays. No more religious school. No more cleaning up for my Dad in the shop. No more getting hit if I didn't do it quite right. Just the teachers getting on at me if I hadn't done my homework. Then three weeks ago, my Dad says this bombshell. I've got to go back to India to get married. His brother has found a man for me. I don't know who he is, not his name even. They just say he's very nice. When I ask how old he is they won't tell me, so I think he must be quite old. Probably about thirty. Mind, I should have known this was going to happen. My cousin it happened to. Now she's living in X (town 80 miles away) with this man she doesn't like and his family and she has to do all the housework and clean the shop and she's the same age as me. She's always on the phone. My Dad doesn't like me talking to her, but he can't stop me. So what to do. I thought of taking loads of tablets just to show them how pissed off I was. That's what my cousin did. It didn't do her any good'.

Thirteen-year-old Hannah: 'What is my life like at the moment? It's good. It's very good. People think because I've got spina bif. and I'm in a wheelchair I must be dead miserable. But I think my life's pretty good. I've got loads of friends at school. My friends all like to push me and the school has got ramps so it's never a problem. I do go to discos on Saturdays. My friends take me. One or two of them will always sit and chat while the others are dancing. So I don't feel left out. I don't think I would want to dance anyway even if it wasn't for this. Some of my friends don't dance and there's nothing wrong with them. Some of the boys used to tease me at primary school. They used to call me 'spastic' and 'mental', but they don't do that now. That really did used to upset me. One of them even said 'Don't you wish you'd never been born, looking like that?' Well, I'm very glad I was born. I'm glad I'm me. I wish he had never been born. Stupid git. I haven't started my periods yet, but me and my Mum, we've worked out what to do. The lady at the Clinic talked to us about it. She wanted to talk about sex too, but I wasn't interested in that'.

Fifteen-year-old Thomas: 'What is my life like at the moment? Rotten really, to be honest. You know I've got cystic fibrosis? Well, I have. I've had it since I was born. It means I'm going to die soon. Well, when I'm about thirty. That's when my older brother died. My Mum wasn't going to have any more, and then I came along. I think I was a bit of a surprise. My Mum was 41 and I think she thought she was past it. It's a laugh. I'm supposed to be in a good phase now and it's true I haven't had to go into hospital for about two years. But I have to take all these tablets and have physio. My Mum does it in the morning and in the evening to drain my chest. It's a real bore. School's boring too. Teachers are daft. Give you a boring lesson and then give you homework on it to make it even more boring. I did have a friend I made at the Clinic. A couple of years older than me. But then he died about six months ago. It really upset me. I couldn't talk to anyone about it. I think my Mum did want to talk about it, but really all she said was that he had cystic fibrosis worse than me and the same wasn't going to happen to me, and I know that's not true.

I don't have a friend now. My Dad just goes off to the pub with his mates. Me and Mum watch television every night and sometimes we get a video. She smokes a lot and I'm not allowed to smoke because of my lungs. She's tried to give it up but she can't. No, I'm not having a great life at the moment, thank you very much'.

These stories are obviously very different, one from another. Indeed, apart from the fact that the young people telling them are all in their teenage years, they seem to have virtually nothing in common. One might ask, does adolescence really exist? Or are there several sorts of adolescence?

1.3 The different ages of puberty

So those in their teens are very different from each other in the lives they lead. As we shall see in more detail in Chapter 6, the differences in the ages when the physical changes of puberty occur mean that they are also very different from each other in the way they look. In girls, as a result of the increase in hormone secretion, changes in the appearance of the shape of the breasts (the first physical sign of puberty) begin at any time between 8 and 13 years with the appearance of the 'breast bud'.

In boys, testosterone levels begin to rise at around 10 years and then rise sharply to reach adult levels. But this can occur at any time between 12 and 17 years. The scrotum and testes begin to enlarge and the scrotum darkens between 11 and 16 years, and the penis grows slightly later to attain adult size on average at any age between 12 and 17 years. In both boys and girls, what is so striking then about the teen years is the great variation in the ages when the physical changes of puberty occur. And comparisons are inevitable. In school, where the young spend so much of their lives, they are very strictly age-segregated. So comparisons with others of the same age are inevitable, as well as being sometimes rather gratifying and sometimes painful. Clearly therefore when it comes to the physical changes of puberty, there is no such thing as a typical 'normal' 13- or 14-year-old.

1.4 The media view of the teenager

The fact that there is no such person as a 'typical' teenager has not stopped the media from projecting images of one. In the first episode of Harry Enfield's television series 'How to be a teenager', Kevin, the prototype for all teenagers, is 6 minutes off his thirteenth birthday. He seems a nice, quiet lad. His mother and father begin to count down the last minutes and then seconds. Ten ... nine ... eight ... three ... two ... one ... zero. There is a small explosion and Kevin the Teenager is born: moody, untidy, rude, disobedient, his face peppered with facial acne. There follow eight years of appalling behaviour. At the other end of his teens, Kevin suddenly emerges as a reasonable human being again. The message is clear. Men may be from Mars and women from Venus, but teenagers arrive direct from Hades.

His poor parents try hard to be understanding. But their heroic efforts to deal with their son's behaviour are futile. They might as well try to understand Einstein's 'Theory of Relativity' or Stephen Hawking's 'Brief History of Time'. Their patience is never rewarded. Their attempts to be friendly are met with contempt. His taste in music and clothes appears to them as bizarre as it is beyond their comprehension. And when they stand their ground on the rules they have made, Kevin is surprised and puzzled. 'It's so unfair', is his constant gripe.

In contrast, here is an account of a very different boy who has just entered the teen years.

John is a 14-year-old boy living with his parents and his 17-year-old sister, Joanna, in a three bedroom house in the suburbs of a city in the Midlands. The home is kept unusually clean and tidy because John's mother is a house-proud woman, who dislikes any sort of mess in the place. It is a family joke that if other members of the family leave books, clothes, or newspapers lying around they can never find them again because she has always tidied them up and put them in places where they can never be discovered. John is pretty much of a conformist and sees himself as a middle of the road teenager, who does not want to stick out in any way. He does averagely well in school, which he does not find particularly interesting, but he has two good mates there whom he likes seeing and kicks a ball about with during breaks. He is not in trouble at school and never has been.

From an early age, John has been quite strong-willed at home where he has always wanted to have his way and found it difficult to accept refusal. There is a family story that when he was only three years old he wanted to go on a dodgem car at a fair with his sister, who had been allowed to drive one. His parents thought he was too young and refused. He cried inconsolably for four hours despite being given other treats and offers of rides with his father. But, in contrast to this experience, throughout his life, John has always been given a say in family decisions, especially if they affect him. Where to go on family holidays, what sort of video to buy, how to redecorate the living room—these sorts of decisions have involved both him and his sister from the time they could understand what was being talked about. John's views have not always won the day, but he has usually felt he has been listened to seriously.

About three months ago, John began to take an interest in a girl of his age in the same class at school, and she in him. She had had a previous boyfriend, while for John this was his first real girlfriend. She was allowed to go out to parties at the weekend until two or three in the morning, and John's parents wanted him home by eleven. They thought he was too young to be out later than that. John's experience of negotiating with his parents helped him to extend his permission up to midnight, but this wasn't enough for his girlfriend who dropped him. John was upset for about a week, and grumpy with his parents whom he tended to blame for his loss. But at no time did he complain about the hour he was expected to be home by. After about a fortnight he had settled down to the idea that he wasn't going to have a girlfriend for a bit.

1.5 **Real teenagers**

So who is the typical teenager, Harry Enfield's Kevin or John in the vignette that I have just described? All the evidence we have from findings from surveys and studies in the UK, USA, Australia, Canada, and the Netherlands is that there is no such thing as a *typical* teenager. As the self-descriptions given earlier in this chapter make clear, those in their teens are extraordinarily different from each other. But boys in their teen years chosen at random from the rest of the population, are much more likely to show features of John than of Kevin. In contrast to Kevin, John's transformation from childhood into an adolescent takes place relatively smoothly. His personality in his teen years is strongly predictable from the way he behaved in childhood earlier in his life.

John's disagreements with his parents are real enough, but they are sorted out without enduring acrimony embittering his relationships with them. He has had these disagreements since he was a young child, and they have shown some increase in his mid-teen years. They have usually been resolved within a few minutes and always within a day or two. Sure enough, there is a generation gap. John's taste in music, clothes, and hairstyle is way different from that of his parents as was theirs from their parents. But John's parents expect this and indeed would be rather worried if he was keener on the popular music of the seventies when they were in their teens than that of his own teenage generation.

Unlike Kevin, John is not particularly moody, disobedient, or rude. Indeed, his behaviour has shown improvement as he has grown into his teen years. He is untidy, but then he always has been. Most important to his parents is that he remains affectionate to them and, although his friends are increasingly significant in his life, he still looks to his parents for advice. He turns to his father when he is short of money or is trying to make up his mind about a purchase, and to his mother when he is in difficulties getting on with his friends. He has, in fact, correctly identified the strengths and weaknesses of each of his parents.

1.6 **The myths, the stereotypes, and the reality**

The fact that there is no such thing as a typical adolescent has not prevented a large number of myths growing up around them. These myths are not just in comedy programmes, like those of Harry Enfield. Both the tabloids and the broadsheets subscribe to them. In mid-2002, BBC Science radio and television programmes were still suggesting there was evidence for them. Yet when they are examined and compared to the available information, it turns out that they have very little substance. For example, in 1992, a psychiatrist, John Offer and an educationist, Kimberley Schonert-Reichl, described some of these myths and then systematically demolished them one by one. The list of myths they produced is far from complete. Here I shall first briefly discuss those that are considered at greater length in later chapters. I shall then go on to discuss other myths at greater length.

Myth No. 1. Normal adolescent development is tumultuous. Those in their teen years are moody, prone to mood swings (at one moment in the depths of despair and the next elated), easily upset, and sensitive to criticism. They are especially likely to have desperate suicidal ideas, and indeed to kill themselves more commonly than adults. In fact, as we shall see in Chapter 4, while puberty does bring with it a more intense emotional life, though mild degrees of moodiness are more common, only about 1 in 10 young people in their teens have violent mood swings. The rate of suicide is lower than that in later life. Temper outbursts are at their peak at about two years and then gradually decline during childhood. They have more or less disappeared as a regular occurrence by mid-adolescence or around the age of 14 years, though, of course, it is not unknown for fully grown adults to lose their tempers when faced with frustration.

Myth No. 2. The teen years are marked by an upsurge of aggression. There are violence peaks during this phase of life. Those in their teens rapidly lose control and are particularly poor at coping calmly with frustration. This topic is considered in more detail in Chapter 5. Most of those in their teens do not show significantly aggressive behaviour. The tendency to hit out when frustrated gradually but very steadily declines during the whole of childhood from the second year of life onwards. Nor does uncontrolled aggression stop at the end of the teens. As shown by government criminal statistics, offences involving violence against the person are more commonly committed by those over 21 (56%) than by those under 21 (44%).

Myth No. 3. Adolescents are obsessed with sex because they are suddenly flooded with sex hormones that drive them into sexual promiscuity. While adults have got sex into proper proportion, adolescents are hormone-driven into thinking about little else. They have the highest rates of unwanted pregnancies resulting in abortion. As we shall see in Chapter 6, while of course an interest in sexual matters greatly increases with puberty, there is no evidence that those in their teens have higher hormone levels than they do in later adulthood. Many adults, especially men, at least until they reach their sixties have sexual thoughts several times a day. Only a minority of those in their teens are sexually promiscuous. Those in their twenties have, on average, more sexual partners. The rate of abortion for unwanted pregnancies is higher in the twenties than it is in the teens.

Myth No. 4. The teen years are inevitably a time of violent disagreement between parents and their children. There is tension between parents and their children, and a tussle for authority. Parents want to hang onto their young; teenagers want to get away from the stranglehold of family life, but at the same time to cling to the love and protection of their parents. Violent conflict inevitably ensues. As we shall see in Chapters 3 and 5, parents and their teenage children generally get on well throughout the teen years. There is an increase in daily hassles, minor disagreements about everyday matters, but these are usually ultimately settled in a friendly manner without long-term rancour. Violent arguments are not the rule, though of course they occur. Emotional separation from parents usually begins in childhood and continues in the teen years. But at the end of the teen years, most young people and their parents remain emotionally attached to each other, and continue to be so later in life. As we shall see, normal development during the teen years does not involve massive parent-child conflict. In fact, the better young people get on with their parents, the better the relationships they make with others of their own age.

Myth No. 5. Those in their teen years, although they may appear superficially clever, are immature in their thinking processes when compared to adults. They see moral dilemmas in black and white terms rather than in more subtle and appropriate ways. There are many different ways of looking at intelligence. Here I shall consider just a few and discuss how those in their teens compare to those in later life.

> *Fluid intelligence* refers to the *processes* of thinking and reasoning. This does indeed gradually improve throughout childhood and reaches maturity in the early teen years. We do not get any better at working out abstract problems we have not met before after the age of 14 or 15 years. For example, two American psychologists looked at 24 subjects in each of four age groups, 9, 14, 18, and 21 years. They tested their competence to make informed treatment decisions in a series of medical dilemmas, involving conditions such as epilepsy, diabetes, and psychological problems.

The children, adolescents, and young adults were given the nature of the problem, alternative treatments, expected benefits, possible risks, and consequences of failure, and then assessed on how much they understood. The 14-year-olds did as well as the 21-year-olds. The 9-year-olds grasped some of the issues, but not others. The authors conclude that 14-year-olds should be treated like adults when it comes to giving consent to medical procedures on themselves. There are a number of similar studies that make it clear that when young people of 13–14 years are compared with young adults in their performance on a task requiring abstract reasoning, so long as neither group has any experience, and both groups are, so to speak, naïve to the task involved, 14-year-olds perform as well as young adults.

Crystallized intelligence refers to the amount people know. This increases as people get older, and then normally declines very slowly indeed as memory begins to fail, or the crystals begin to flake a little! The crystals may take quite a time to flake. In one study psychologists found that 19-year-old college students were not as good at general knowledge questions as a group of older people with an average age of 79 years! So crystalline intelligence (what we know), does not stop accumulating after early adolescence. Nor indeed does it ever stop accumulating. Many 80-year-olds have succeeded in learning a foreign language for the first time, and each year the Open University awards degrees to people of this age who have successfully completed a demanding course of study. The concept of lifelong learning requires the ability to acquire knowledge throughout life.

Street cred; another type of intelligence. Obviously older people do know more than adolescents in those many areas of life in which they have had more experience and in knowledge learned from books. But there are plenty of life skills in which adolescents have more experience than adults. Many school teachers responsible for drug education recognize that there are quite a few teenagers around who know more about ways of obtaining drugs, the different experiences you can expect from using them, and possible harmful side effects than they do themselves. If I wanted to know which streets in a rough part of London to avoid so as not to get mugged, I would expect to get a more accurate answer from a local teenager than from an older local resident.

Wisdom: another type of intelligence. All the same, we should be cautious about accepting the notion that thinking processes do not improve after early adolescence even though such improvement may be very difficult to measure. The reasoning powers shown by mathematicians or literary critics in their thirties or forties may represent a major advance from those they have shown in adolescence, not just in what they know but also in how they process knowledge. The same may be said of decision-making involving the use of judgement, the bringing together of reason with experience. As Robert Sternberg has put it, there are not all that many 'wise' adolescents walking around, but there are quite a few older people who are thought of as wise.

Myth No. 6. The teen years form a separate phase of life. This period of life is clearly separated from both childhood and adulthood. We are right to treat those in their teens differently from everyone else because they are indeed different from the rest of the population. Harry Enfield's Kevin is transformed from a child to an adolescent virtually instantaneously. Further, he abruptly reverts from teenage monster to a normal human being when he reaches the end of his teen years. In fact, the great majority of young people do not show an abrupt transformation of this type either at the beginning or at the end of the teen years. The behaviour of most adolescents is quite recognizable from their behaviour in childhood; there is much stability between adolescence and young adulthood. This is not to claim that teenagers like Kevin do not exist. Of course they do and they make brilliant subjects for television programmes, but they convey a highly misleading and, if one takes them seriously, a highly derogatory message about the teen years.

In fact, the teen years have extremely fuzzy edges. Well before puberty begins, many children of 9–11 years, if not earlier, are showing an interest in sexy clothes, erotic music, and having friends of the opposite sex, boyfriends or girlfriends, behaving indeed in much the same way as those in their teens. So-called 'tweenagers' or 'tweenies' are now targeted in most western European and north American countries by those marketing clothes and popular music. Many parents spend considerable sums of money to keep their pre-teen children in fashion. Whatever the 'tweenager' phenomenon is due to, and most believe that the sexualization of the pre-teen years is manufactured by commercial interests, the fact is that the beginning of adolescence is far from clear-cut. Indeed this has always been the case. The change is merely that the blurred lines are occurring earlier.

The same blurring occurs at the end of the teen years. The idea of the teens as a halfway stage between childhood and adulthood, ending at the end of the teens, is not confirmed by the views of parents or, very clearly, what young people think about themselves. An American study carried out by Jeffrey Jensen Arnett from the University of Maryland has shown that most people aged between 18 and 25 years are uncertain whether by that age they have reached adulthood. Three in five of people aged 18–25 years say 'Yes and No' in answer to the question, 'Do You Feel You Have Reached Adulthood'?

Only two in five say 'Yes'. Interestingly, nearly one in two young people aged 12–17 years also say 'Yes and No' in answer to the same question, so there is little shift between the two age groups. Both age groups are uncertain whether they have reached adulthood. Arnett believes there is a phase of life he calls 'Emerging Adulthood' from 18 to 25 years that is neither adolescence nor adulthood. He describes this period as one of exploration in relationships and work, in which the so-called 'risk behaviours' are at their peak. It sounds extraordinarily like the popular view of adolescence to me.

When we look at this belief that there is a clear separation between childhood and adolescence and between adolescence and adult life in other ways, we find it is equally misleading. As we saw earlier in this chapter, although the early teen years are certainly of importance in physical sexual development, in many children a great deal happens before they start and most of the action is over by the time the teens are halfway completed. What about other aspects of physical development?

The development of the brain. If the teens really were a separate phase of life, one would expect changes in the brain to occur when it starts and to stop when it finishes. This just does not occur. The brain reaches its adult weight some years after birth but before puberty. However, many important changes in the brain occur well after birth and some indeed continue into adult life. Nerve cells or neurones continue to migrate from the place they first appear to their final site in the brain for some years after birth. New synapses, or connections between neurones, are formed over this time. A substance called myelin forms a sheath around nerve cells and is important for the rapid conduction of nerve impulses along the nerves. New myelin is laid down during the whole of childhood, and this continues well into adolescence and at least into the early twenties, possibly longer. A large number of superfluous nerve cells and connections are made during fetal life and in the first two years of life. This means that for greater efficiency of brain function it is necessary for a large number of gray matter cells to die and for the 'architecture' of the brain to be gradually moulded into a mature form. Some of these changes accelerate in the pre-teen years and continue through the teen years well into the twenties. There is no reason to think, as Barbara Rausch has suggested in her condescendingly entitled book about teenagers 'Why Are They So Weird?' that the adolescent brain is different and that this explains the chaotic emotional life of the teenager. As most young people of this age do not experience emotional chaos, there is no need to develop theories about brain function to explain it. The same changes in brain development occur in children and young people all over the world. As we shall see in the next chapter, the variation in behaviour between cultures is enormous. It is society that creates our teenagers, not their brains.

Different ways of thinking do not suddenly appear in the early teens. The teenage capacity to think in abstract terms does not suddenly arrive out of nowhere. In the last two decades of the twentieth century, it has been shown that abstract thinking is present to some degree in younger children and that the process of achieving it is continuous from childhood through to adolescence. Psychologists such as Daniel Keating have pointed to the gradual way in which these capacities are acquired. Bearing in mind the lack of evidence for any sudden underlying change in the brain at adolescence, it does seem more likely that this is the case.

This fits in with our observations of younger children, especially when they are really gripped by a problem. After all, fairness is an abstract idea. But it is not at all uncommon to hear 8-year-olds complain of being victims of unfairness, and they use the word, quite appropriately, in an adult way—they think they have been hard done by. Motivation is another abstract idea. Yet many 8-year-olds seem quite capable of accepting the idea that a goalkeeper's motivation is in question and might be difficult to judge with certainty. 'He wasn't really trying', is an idea well within the average 8-year-old's capacity to understand. On the other hand, one would not expect a child of this age to be able to tolerate uncertainty. Was the striker deliberately fouled by the goalkeeper? Younger children would have difficulty accepting that it just is not possible to know even by studying the video clip, and that perhaps even the goalkeeper himself is not quite sure. By the age of around 12–13 years, this is no longer a problem.

Myth No. 7. Adolescents have constant doubts about their identity. Characteristically they show uncertainty about who they are, why they have been born, what they are going to do in life, how they compare with others of their own age, and how physically attractive they are. They are in trouble if they have not sorted out all these uncertainties by the end of adolescence. The development of identity provides perhaps the greatest claim of adolescence and the teen years to a very special status in psychological development. The conventional wisdom is that it is only in the teen years that individuals ask themselves ' Who am I'? 'What sort of a person am I'? But how well does this belief that adolescence is crucial to the development of identity stand up to scrutiny?

The claim arises originally from the work of Erik Eriksen in the 1950s and 1960s. He suggested that to be fully mature, an individual had to have a sense of ego identity, an idea or set of ideas of ourselves that is enduring, and continuous over time. According to Eriksen, there is a personal identity, consisting of one's values and aspirations and a social identity deriving from the many roles one may play in life, for example as worker, father, son, wife, friend, sportsman.

Adolescence is the time, he wrote, when it is crucial that a unique adult personal identity with a meaningful role in life is formed.

Eriksen suggested there was only one desirable route to the achievement of such a mature identity. This involved a period of exploration and experimentation during the teen years. During this period there should be a ban or 'moratarium' on premature establishment of identity. Exploration could result in an enormous amount of self-questioning, and this might quite normally amount to an 'identity crisis'. During this crisis, the adolescent would need to make some clear decisions about her values, the sort of person she wanted to be, and the sort of life she wanted to lead. A clear personal and social identity should emerge. But as well as this achievement of a mature identity, there were two undesirable outcomes. Adolescents might make up their minds too quickly and land up with an identity that didn't suit their personalities. This was called 'foreclosure'. Alternatively, they might never emerge from their period of exploration and drift forever uncertain of their identity. This unsatisfactory state of mind was called 'identity diffusion'.

Eriksen's ideas have been widely elaborated as well as criticized since the time he formulated them. It has been pointed out that he expresses a notion of identity that involves a form of personal integrity, unrelated to the wishes and needs of other people. But for most people, especially for most girls and women and preferably also for most boys and men, personal identity involves not just meeting one's own needs, but also responding to the needs of others. It has also been powerfully argued that Eriksen's concept of the development of identity implies that the individual is free to choose his or her identity, whereas in the real world, the idea one has of oneself is heavily influenced by social class, gender, and ethnic group. Increasingly, identity, especially in young people, is seen to emerge from their lifestyle, the sort of friends they mix with, the sort of music they enjoy, the clothes they buy, and the way they spend their evenings and weekends. It seems reasonable to think that lifestyle influences identity just as identity influences lifestyle.

But there is another, more powerful criticism that needs to be made. Eriksen firmly placed the task of identity formation exclusively in the adolescent or teen years. In fact, identity development begins in the early years of life. From the time, and typically this is around the age of two and a half years, a boy comes to realize he is like other boys and not like a girl, his identity formation has begun. As he enters school for the first time at the age of four or five years, he will begin to think of himself as being clever or not so clever, good or not so good at sport. Towards the end of his primary school days, he may well begin to think of his career after he leaves school or higher education. At this point, his work or career identity will be strongly influenced by his social class.

During his teen years his identity formation will certainly continue. Beliefs and values, often derived from a mixture of parents and admired friends, will be formed and may superficially seem established, but identity formation does not stop at the end of adolescence as Eriksen suggested it did. Beliefs and values can change throughout life and identity formation continues well into adult life and beyond.

The single, unattached girl will have a different identity at twenty-two from that she experiences at twenty-five when she has a regular boyfriend. The man behaving badly at thirty something may have quite different ideas about himself and his future five years later when he has a wife and a young child. In the post-modern world, the 40-year-old furnace worker who has a view of himself as a man who earns his living by his brawn and muscle power, may think very differently when he has been made redundant, has retrained, and is now working as a computer programmer. The 50-year-old woman, emerging from the break-up of her marriage and looking to make a new intimate relationship will find herself coping with many of the identity issues she had thought she had left behind at eighteen. 'Who am I'? once again becomes an important question for her. Indeed she may rather resent anyone who suggests she is behaving 'like an adolescent'. The man who has retired at sixty but feels full of energy, may need to carve out a new identity for himself in voluntary work or on the golf course, or perhaps both.

The development of identity is a lifelong task. It probably stops only on one's death bed when one asks oneself what sort of a life one has had and what sort of a death one is capable of making. Throughout the whole of life, part of one's identity has involved an idea of the sort of a job one can make of dying. Now, with experience, this part of one's identity may change. Of course the teen years are a time when identity changes occur, but it is by no means the time of life when personal identity is developed and established once and for all. Much has gone on before and even more will go on afterwards. Formation of our identities goes on for the whole of life.

Myth No. 8. Those in their teen years are emotionally immature. It is often said about those in their teen years that everything happens too quickly for them. Their bodies are developing earlier; they have earlier sexual experience and adult lifestyles in their drinking and drug-taking. But they cannot cope emotionally with all these experiences. Even though they may be physically well developed, they are emotionally immature.

How emotionally mature are adolescents? Emotional maturity is a very vague term, but we do know a great deal about different aspects of emotional development throughout the teen years. Essential components of emotional maturity include the capacity to avoid giving way to immediate impulses, avoidance of situations that would be too difficult to handle, and the ability to deal with frustration without losing emotional control. All the evidence suggests that these develop throughout childhood and continue to improve throughout adolescence. The 18-year-old can certainly handle emotionally demanding situations a great deal better than a 13-year-old.

It is therefore not a myth that those in their early teens are much less emotionally mature than those in their late teens. But we need to consider why this should be. Is this ineptitude of the 13-year-old inevitable, perhaps a result of immaturity of the brain? Or does it arise from the fact that 13-year-olds are not adequately prepared for the emotionally demanding experiences they may encounter? All the evidence suggests it arises because of the lack of adequate preparation.

Having worked in a children's hospital dealing with the most serious children's illnesses, I have not infrequently seen young people in their early teens who have faced what must surely be one of the most testing emotional experiences of all, the loss of a much loved younger brother or sister. If they have been well prepared by their parents and supported by nursing and medical staff, they have dealt with this situation emotionally remarkably well. Of course, they have been deeply upset, but they have usually shown considerable capacity to come through the ordeal intact as well as to provide great support and comfort to their grieving parents. Again, if they are well prepared, young people of this age show remarkable ability to control their anger in the face of extreme provocation. Of course, when younger brothers or sisters take their belongings or tease them mercilessly, some of those in their teens do react angrily, but most manage to keep their cool and deal with the situation in a mature manner. In Chapter 3, I describe the tens of thousands of the so-called 'young carers', another group of young people who, given some help, cope remarkably well when circumstances, especially the illness of their parents, force them to take unusual levels of responsibility.

At any age, it is experience that matures us emotionally. If we are well prepared for emotionally challenging experiences, such maturation will occur all the more smoothly. If those in their teen years are expected to face new experiences in ignorance and confusion, without adequate support, like people of any age they will mess up their own lives as well as those of others. So, unlike all the other myths I have considered, the belief that those in their teens are emotionally immature is not a false belief. But it is largely true not because of any intrinsic failure of those in their teens, but because of the inadequate way they are prepared for emotionally stressful situations. In Chapter 9, I shall consider how better preparation involving the promotion of so-called 'emotional intelligence' might greatly change the situation.

In any case, it would be wrong to suggest that most of those in their teens currently lack the ability to keep out of situations they cannot handle or control their emotions or that, as a group, they lack empathy or sympathy. As family relationships change with an increase in autonomy, it is often the teenager, in touch with his parents' feelings of anxiety about 'letting go' who brings his parents through this stage successfully rather than the other way round. All the same, there is a significant minority for whom emotional immaturity is a major liability. Those in their teens who are temperamentally vulnerable, or who have suffered abuse and other forms of trauma will indeed be at serious risk as a result of their inability to resist the temptations that are offered to young people, even if they have been well prepared for their experiences. To generalise from them to all teenagers would be a serious mistake.

Myth No. 9. Those in their teens are characteristically full of naïve idealism. They latch on to social causes, undergo religious conversions, develop attachments to extremist political parties, and take up global issues such as environmental pollution and global warming in a completely unrealistic manner. They rapidly lose their idealism once they enter adult life and face the 'real world'. Of course, some of those in their teens are unrealistically optimistic about their capacity to change the world. But most of these activities or beliefs are much more a feature of the early and mid-twenties than of the teen years. The twenties is the age when people most actively campaign for environmental improvements and join extremist political or religious movements. Though fortunately some young people in their teens are indeed idealistic in their views, many are extremely 'hard-nosed' in their attitude to the world and their own future, choosing career options that they think will give them steady jobs and/or make them high earners. Nor do those in their teens and twenties have a monopoly of idealism. Numerous people retain a sense of idealism throughout their lives. It is notable that those who remain idealistic are often referred to as 'adolescent', the word then being used as an insult, to imply they have never properly grown up. When this happens, an entire phase of life is maligned and, at the same time, those valuable people who are vital for the support of many worthwhile but politically difficult causes are condemned.

Myth No. 10. The teens have the greater abundance of creativity and new ideas. This is just not true. When one looks at the maximum periods of creativity of great artists, even those such as Mozart and Picasso who have been extraordinarily productive in their teens, reached greater inventive heights later in their lives. More systematic tests of different types of intelligence do show that the peak of our creativity and the capacity to innovate are reached earlier than many other capacities, but the level reached in the teens is nearly always maintained well into adult life. Even in those fields such as mathematics where most new work is carried out in early life, the period of maximum achievement is usually in the twenties and only occasionally in the teens.

1.7 **Why have these myths persisted?**

In the next chapter, I shall discuss the ways in which the myths I have described have arisen in more detail. Here I just want to point out that one of the reasons for their wide currency is the fact that, for a relatively small minority of young people in their teens, they are not myths at all, but factually accurate beliefs. There are indeed young people of this age who are moody, suicidal, violently aggressive, academically weak, sexually promiscuous, and emotionally extremely immature. These are the young people who figure prominently in the media.

Those in their teens can be divided into three groups: the non-problematic conformists (the majority), the non-problematic non-conformists (a conspicuous minority), and the problematic minority. We know, with some certainty because this is the group those who conduct surveys are really interested in, that about one in five fall into the problematic group. It isn't meaningful to estimate the size of the other two groups, because so often young people drift from one group to another during the teen years.

The good news for parents is, of course, that four out of five teenage children are neither unusually troubled nor troubling. Indeed, though at times they may be irritating, outrageous, and unpredictable, on balance their parents are likely to regard them as a source of pleasure and delight.

All the same, the fact that as many as one in five young people in their teens have significant problems is a cause for serious concern. Such problems mainly consist of disturbed emotions, especially depression, anxiety, and anorexia; or disruptive behaviour; or a mixture of these. As we shall see in Chapter 4, those with disturbed emotions are not showing trivial upset. They sometimes suffer so deeply they may attempt, or even very occasionally commit, suicide. They may starve themselves to a worrying degree, again, very, very occasionally to the point of death. The disruptive group, as we shall see in Chapter 5, not only affect their own lives but the lives of others, sometimes making school classrooms places where useful learning just cannot occur no matter how good the teacher. They may completely ruin the lives of elderly people whom they terrorize. So it is not a myth that a small proportion of those in their teens are deeply disturbed and disturbing. It is a very worrying truth. But it is a complete travesty of the truth to label the majority of those in this phase of life with such a reputation. Every age group has a troubled and troublesome minority; the teens are no exception.

1.8 **The stigmatization of the teen phase of life**

Earlier in this chapter, we have seen how myths about adolescence abound and how misleading they are. In the next chapter, I shall attempt to show how they have arisen over time. The fact is that those in their teen years are stigmatized. They experience the negative effects from which all stigmatized groups suffer. A stigma is a mark of shame and humiliation that brands individuals because they belong to a group regarded as inferior. Discrimination involves making distinctions or preferences that have the effect of producing social exclusion or disadvantage.

Anyone who observed about a bad driver 'What do you expect, she's a woman' or who said of an elderly person who seemed confused 'What do you expect, she's just old' would soon be pulled up. Not just by the obsessionally politically correct, but by most ordinary people. Yet if you see a badly behaved teenager and say 'What do you expect, he's adolescent' there will be no such protest. The word is frequently used to describe the irresponsible, the thoughtless, the selfish. When divorced or separated people experiment with different relationships before settling down to a single partner, they are often described in a dismissive way as 'behaving just like adolescents'. In fact, they are behaving like most sexually mature people do when they are without a regular partner.

Much, though doubtless not enough, improvement was made during the second half of the twentieth century in the degree to which women (especially those pursuing careers), ethnic minority groups, the mentally ill, the learning disabled, and the elderly are discriminated against. A necessary condition for such improvement has been the recognition both of the fact and of the unfairness of stigmatization. Such recognition has not yet happened as far as those in their teens are concerned. Before real change comes about, there needs to be greater awareness of what is happening to them.

In the chapters that follow, I shall discuss how adolescents have suffered from the stigmatization that comes from stereotyping in their education, their family relationships, their leisure activities, their sexual activities, in the expectation they will show criminal behaviour, in attitudes to their use of drugs and alcohol, and in their political exclusion. In each of these areas, the separation and segregation of adolescents from the rest of society and the myths about them have resulted in harm not just to those in their teens themselves, but to all of us.

The teen years in western society today, at the beginning of the twenty-first century are a poor preparation for the rest of life. Young people of this age, while extraordinarily diverse in their behaviour and competence, are too frequently over-protected and infantilized by a society that fails to recognize what most of them can do if given the opportunity. The sense of a 'generation apart', of the alienation of a whole segment of our population that has been led to believe it is much more immature than in fact it need be, cannot be good for adolescents or for the rest of us.

A change is now detectable. Over the last decade of the twentieth century, the stereotype of the immature adolescent began to weaken. But much of the adult population, reinforced by the media, continue to see adolescents as either generally incompetent and vulnerable or wielding power they cannot control. At the same time, changes are occurring in the way we think of those in their teen years, in the way we expect them to behave and indeed in the way they are behaving. In general, although there is sometimes quite strong resistance to these new ideas, especially, as one might expect, from those who stand to lose most if they gain currency, there is encouraging evidence of a transformation of adolescence. New, altogether more competent adolescents are emerging. We should welcome them into the twenty-first century.

In the next chapter, I shall try to show how the stereotype of the weak, incompetent adolescent arose in historical times and how the adult world manufactures the adolescents it needs. I then go on in subsequent chapters to discuss different aspects of the way those in their teen years function in the world that has been manufactured for them in western society today. In the last chapter, I suggest ways in which policy makers are already making the world they live in a place more likely to allow them to exercise the competence of which they are capable, and to suggest other approaches to this desirable outcome.

Messages for parents and teachers.

- Those in their teen years live extraordinarily varied lives, depending on their circumstances.

- There is no sharp beginning or end to adolescence. There are blurred boundaries between childhood and the teen years and between the teen years and adulthood.

- From historical times, those in their teens have always had a bad image and continue to do so today.

- The stereotyped but incorrect view of adolescents as immature and incompetent continues to receive approval from some authoritative social scientists and mental health professionals.

- Most young people in their teens do not conform to the stereotypes held by adults about them.

- The negative, disparaging view of teenagers held by adults does them harm and, in the end, harms adults too. Fortunately there are encouraging signs that it is losing its power.

Chapter 2

The invention of adolescence

2.1 The meaning of adolescence

2.1.1 Where the word comes from

The term 'adolescence' was first used in ancient Rome, probably by Plautus, around 193 BC. 'Adolescere' is Latin for 'to grow up' and adultus means 'to have grown up'. So, in a sense, adults are defined in terms of the completion of their adolescence. The term 'adolescent' was used by churchmen and other scholars in classical times and in the Middle Ages to describe young people who had not achieved full adult social rights. This might take a long time and some eminent doctors and churchmen who wrote about the young laid it down that the end of adolescence did not arrive until the age of 35 or even 42 years. But it always began round about the time of the beginning of puberty. In those days this was later than it is today, on average at about 14–15 years.

Towards the end of the Middle Ages, and with the decline in the use of Latin and words derived from Latin, the word adolescence largely went out of use in English speaking countries, and was replaced with the term 'youth'.

2.1.2 'Youth' replaces 'adolescence'

The word 'youth' was not used in the same way as 'adolescence'. It was usually seen to begin before puberty at the time when children began to be gainfully employed. This might happen at the age of seven or eight years. The length of 'youth' depended on when adult status was reached, as shown by marriage or starting self-employment. So a young person who married at twenty would stop being a youth 10 years earlier than one who married at thirty. Mostly the term was used for children and young people from around the age of 10 years up to about the age of 25 years. There was no separate word for teenagers. Young people in their teen years were just seen as in the middle of their period of 'youth'.

2.1.3 The return of adolescence

The term 'youth' continued to be the only term in use to describe the young who had grown beyond childhood until, as we shall see later, the beginning of the twentieth century. Following the publication of a weighty work written by an American philosopher, psychologist, and educationist, G. Stanley Hall, psychologists started to use the word 'adolescence', the title of Hall's book. At this point, the idea of adolescence entered the artistic world. Part 2 of Stravinsky's Rites of Spring, titled 'Dance of the Adolescents' with its thumping sexual rhythms, written in 1912, and Edvard Munch's painting 'Adolescence' of the same period, portraying a frail, vulnerable girl in her mid-teens, reflected two contrasting, artistic expressions of the same subject. In its revived form, adolescence was now more narrowly defined as the teen years and has continued to be used in this way for the last hundred years.

2.1.4 'Teenagers' appear'

In the early 1940s, the term 'teenager' appeared for the first time, probably in an article published in an American magazine, *Popular Science*, in 1941. It is thought to have leaked into the language from the world of advertising. To create a youth market it was thought to be desirable to define those in the teen years as having special consumer needs. People in this age group would be given an exciting sense of identity that would be attractive to them. They would want to belong to it and would buy whatever was necessary to make them feel part of it. From then on, marketing directors, journalists, the general public, and indeed those in the teen years themselves have much preferred the term 'teenager'. The terms 'youth' and 'adolescence' are now mainly used by professionals and academics, though in the UK the youth sector and the Youth Service cater to the needs of the 12 to 25s.

2.2 Ideas of youth and where they come from

2.2.1 The young have always had a bad press

In historical times, as we have seen, at least up to the middle of the nineteenth century, the teen years were not seen as a separate phase of life, but as a part of what was called 'youth' stretching from around puberty or even a year or two beforehand until the time of marriage in the case of girls or marriage and independent employment in boys and young men. 'Youth' was generally written about disparagingly. Aristotle, in the 4th century BC, wrote, 'The young are in character prone to desire and ready to carry any desire they have into action. Of bodily desires it is the sexual to which they are most disposed to give way, and in regard to sexual desire they exercise no self-restraint. They are changeful too, and fickle in their desires … passionate, irascible, and apt to be carried away by their impulses'. Two millennia later, William Shakespeare put into the mouth of the Old Shepherd in The Winter's Tale the words, 'I would there were no age between ten and three and twenty … for there is nothing in the between but getting wenches with child, wronging the ancientry, stealing, fighting …'.

2.2.2 The sinful teens

In every age the way adolescence has been seen has depended on the prevailing beliefs about the world current at the time. In medieval times and in early modern England, the prevailing ideology was derived from Augustinian theology. The concept of youthful sin was then deeply rooted. As Ilana Krausman Ben-Amos, a historian of youth, puts it, 'mediaeval preachers stressed that human predilection to sin became particularly marked in children who reached seven years, and as they grew up to adolescence and youth, their tendency to sin, to a lack of control over sexual passions, and to indulgence in bodily pleasures grew.' The Renaissance did not bring a change of view. Erasmus believed that 'human instincts tended towards wrongdoing, evil and vice, which were especially marked in infants, children and youth.' In Early Modern England, Protestant preachers after the Reformation confirmed these beliefs. Youths were, by nature, 'brutish and devilish.' Clearly they were quite unsuitable to hold positions of responsibility.

At the same time, alongside such Christian belief and in some respects antedating it, an astrological belief system was a powerful influence. According to the Ptolemaic system, devised in the second century, Venus was the planet guiding the fate of young people aged 14–22 years. This planet 'implanted an impulse towards the embrace of love.' The Seven Ages of Man famously described by Jacques in Shakespeare's 'As You Like It', follow this astrological design. The lovesick youth, his fate guided by the planet Venus, cannot be expected to do much in the world but pine for his lost love.

In fact ideas about young people usually have remarkably little resemblance to how they actually behave. At the same time as the young were in receipt of constant disparagement, not just by opinion leaders of their time such as Aristotle and Shakespeare, but by virtually everyone who wrote about them, their behaviour continued to belie their negative stereotype. For example, at the time Shakespeare was writing, though a high proportion (as many as one in three) of women were pregnant at the time of marriage, the average age of marriage in Elizabethan times was in the mid to late twenties and the rate of illegitimacy was extraordinarily low. Contraception was ineffective at that time, so it is highly unlikely that young people in their teens were promiscuously engaged in sexual intercourse. Nor is there any good evidence for antisocial behaviour as the norm among this age group.

2.2.3 **The Romantic Age**

With the development of Romanticism throughout the western world, the late eighteenth century saw the flowering of the concept of the 'natural' child and youth, pristine and unblemished by contact with a corrupting world. This Rousseauesque vision developed alongside the publication of Goethe's 'Sorrows of Young Werther', a novel describing the neurotic debility of a young man, eventually driven to suicide by grief over his lost love. The wild success of the novel, reinforced the idea that it was 'natural' for youths, or at least those who could afford it, to spend their days and nights in mournful regret for what might have been in their love lives. This state of mind was clearly not conducive to serious employment and the number of suicides in young people increased. The novel was banned in a number of German states.

2.3 **The scientific study of the teen years**

2.3.1 **The evolutionary view: G. Stanley Hall**

Evolutionary theory in the mid-nineteenth century paved the way for the first so-called scientific theories of adolescence. These too provided a justification for a prolonged state of semi-dependency. G. Stanley Hall, in the two volume work 'Adolescence', published in 1904, proposed that the phases of life of an individual could best be understood as a repeat performance of the development of the human race. Thus childhood was an enactment of early, primitive forms of savage existence. Adolescence was 'a new birth, for the higher and more completely human traits are now born .... The child comes from and harks back to a remoter past; the adolescent is neo-atavistic, and in him the later acquisitions of the race slowly become prepotent.' Like Rousseau, Hall saw adolescence as a time of purity and idealism, but also, like many others before and after him, believed that, in his time, the dangers of corruption were greater than ever. 'Never', he wrote 'has youth been exposed to such dangers of both perversion and arrest as in our own land (the United States) and day'.

Hall believed in adolescence as 'naturally', inevitably and appropriately tempestuous, characterized by emotional 'sturm und drang', or storm and stress. The idea that lack of emotional control is an intrinsic part of adolescence inevitably results in immediate disqualification of the whole age group from taking any sort of responsibility for themselves or for others. It is an idea that persisted, especially in the media and in literature, throughout the whole of the twentieth century, nourished initially by Hall, but given a strong further impetus by Freud and his followers in psychoanalysis.

2.3.2 **The psychoanalytic view**

Freud provided a rationale for the supposed, inevitably conflictual, stormy nature of adolescence. Increased sexual arousal reactivated infantile wishes to possess the parent of opposite sex. Forbidden, deeply repressed, unconscious desires resulted in the experience of emotional turbulence until mature sexual relationships with a partner were established. Peter Blos, a prominent American psychoanalyst, wrote, 'The more or less orderly course of development ... is thrown into disarray with the child's entry into adolescence ... adolescence cannot take its normal course without regression.' Freud's daughter, Anna, saw disturbance as a sign of normality—'the upholding of a steady equilibrium during the adolescent process is in itself abnormal.'

Donald Winnicott, an influential British psychoanalyst, seems to have seen adolescence as an illness. He wrote, 'The cure for adolescence belongs to the passage of time and to the gradual maturation process. The crucial thing to be recognised', he added 'is the fact that the adolescent boy or girl do not want to be understood. Adults must hide among themselves what they come to understand of adolescence'. Winnicott, like Freud, saw adolescence as a time when there was a reactivation of infantile sexual problems. As we shall see, this improbable explanation of a non-existent phenomenon was not a satisfactory basis to guide policies for the young. But, for several generations of educationists and professionals dealing with disturbed youngsters and delinquents, psychoanalysis has been and continues to be a powerful influence. Journalists and others writing for the public still assume, as a part of received wisdom, that adolescence is inevitably and naturally a time of emotional crisis. In a BBC One television documentary on the teen years shown in the summer of 2002, an American psychoanalyst said that if he heard of a young person who had passed through the teen years without a significant amount of upset, he would be pretty sure there was a serious mental illness present. Such ideas continue to exist and are as misleading and possibly dangerous as they ever were.

Modern theories of adolescence have been developed over the last 30 years that have more credibility. In view of the discrediting of previous views of adolescence, that may seem improbable. But current scientific views are more broadly and firmly based than their predecessors. They depend on studies of adolescents without problems as well as those with difficulties. They pay greater regard to the adolescent as an active participant in the world around him or her. No longer is the teenager seen as just a passive recipient of influences from the family or from school. There is greater acceptance too of the diversity of adolescent lives and of the fact that young people can readily play different roles depending on what is expected of them. Most importantly, there is greater acceptance of the notion of continuity between childhood and adolescence and between adolescence and adulthood.

During the last years of the twentieth century the social sciences have gradually dispelled the myths surrounding the stereotype of adolescence. But this stereotype persists in the media and is regarded as valid by many who work in this field. In the 1980s, for example, a study was published showing that American mental health professionals viewed normal adolescents as significantly more disturbed than did adolescents themselves. When they were asked to complete a questionnaire about their behaviour as a 'normal, mentally healthy adolescent' might complete it, these professionals described themselves as having all sorts of problems, that it is well established most of those in their teens show quite infrequently.

So even among professionals, out of date ideas about adolescence persist. And this is even truer of the media. New scientific findings make less dramatic reading. The language of crisis, of storm and stress, and the view of the young as powerful, violent, young monsters driven by their sex hormones is much more newsworthy.

2.4 The teens as separate: the brain child of nineteenth century pedagogues

The idea of the teen years as a separate phase of existence began in the first half of the nineteenth century. Although the word 'adolescence' only began to be used in its modern sense of the teen years at the beginning of the twentieth century, the seeds of the idea of separateness of this time of life were sown in the ethos of the large public boarding school.

This was developed initially by Thomas Arnold, Headmaster of Rugby School between 1827 and 1839, and applied specifically to boys in their teen years or at least up to the age of 17 or 18 years when they left school. Arnold's regime and those of other headmasters in large public schools, was developed partly to deal with the violent and chaotic situation that had arisen as a result of cramming boys together away from home and giving them poor education and worse care. Now, in many such schools boys were expected to be clean in body and mind. Soap cleansed the body and moral exhortation, backed by threats of dire punishment for unclean thoughts, the mind. Schoolmasters, backed by orthodox medical opinion, disseminated the view that masturbation caused insanity. There was a strong emphasis on the notion of conformity. Boys who did not step out of line were praised and those who were in any way 'different' were despised. Cleverness was regarded with suspicion and even teachers held strong anti-intellectual values. Athletic ability was held in high esteem, but not if the talented athlete behaved as if he were in any way superior. These values were upheld without fear of contradiction because the school behaved like a 'total institution' isolated from the real world. It had its own hierarchy consisting of a prefectorial system, backed by a system of fagging with servant status for new school entrants.

This 'public school' ethos was applied specifically to boys in their teen years. It was not thought relevant to younger children nor to those entering University where different values prevailed. So a modern, middle class lifestyle, with a prolonged period of education and financial dependency, arose for teenage boys, though not for girls, well before the word 'adolescence' was revived to describe it.

2.5 The life of the middle class young in their teen years 1900–1960

By the end of the nineteenth century the period from 13 to 18 years was being clearly seen by writers and educators as a separate phase of life. The age segregation in schools and the later age of school leaving among middle class children meant that these five or six years were seen as special. 'Adolescence' began with the onset of puberty and ended with school leaving and taking up employment or beginning further study at University. Although the term had been used in France and the United States as much as half a century earlier, the British started to talk about adolescence in the early years of the twentieth century.

It was at this point that adolescence began to be more widely seen as an especially vulnerable period. Moodiness and impulsiveness were seen as characteristic. Inability to control impulses increased the risk of turning to a life of crime at this time. There was increasing concern about the rising crime rate and the increasing size of the prison population, mainly consisting of young people. But instead of seeing crime as arising from poverty, hunger, and overcrowding, as well as from lack of education and regular, reasonably paid employment, it was now viewed as an 'adolescent' phenomenon, something that arose from a badly brought up age group rather than linked more generally to social disadvantage and poverty.

In fact, criminal activity was largely concentrated in the most disadvantaged sections of the population. Even within the worst off areas, as Robert Roberts makes clear in his book 'The Classic Slum', it was the young from the poorest families that attracted prison sentences. Though sometimes serious, often their offences were trivial, involving for example snowballing, playing football, or gambling in the streets. In these districts, violence was rife.

Roberts writes he hardly knew a weekend free from the sight of brawling adults and inter-family disputes.

Life was very different for the young of the middle classes. In contrast to working class young people, middle class children in their teenage years, girls as well as boys, were almost all in full-time school until at least 14 or 15 years and often longer. The compulsory leaving age was raised to 14 years in 1918, at the end of the First World War, but by this time nearly all middle class children were staying on at school longer than this anyway. The same was the case when compulsory school leaving was raised to 15 years in 1945. Schools were now strongly age-segregated, with few or no exceptions made for children who were brighter than the rest or had more learning difficulties. Most pupils of secondary age went to single-sex day schools, whether grammar, public or private, usually church schools. A minority went to public boarding schools or to cheaper private boarding schools. A system of regulation, introduced in 1902, when the secondary school system first became administered by local authorities, resulted in improvement in the quality of schooling, though many schools remained brutal in their methods of instilling discipline, with frequent beating both by masters and prefects. Standards of literacy and numeracy in middle class children were now high.

On leaving school, boys would go into the family firm, the business of a friend of the family, begin training for one of the professions or, in competition with others, find a job in a shop, bank, or small business. Girls stayed at home, became shop assistants or trained to become secretaries. A small number of young men and a much smaller number of young women went on to University.

Whether still at school or at work, social life for the middle class child in his or her teen years revolved around the family. Mothers were the centre of family life and fathers, although the repository of ultimate authority in the family, were likely to be relatively remote figures. Fathers in business worked long hours, usually 50–60 hours a week, at the office, in the shop, or at the bank and this meant many returned home exhausted and uncommunicative. Those in other occupations were also likely to be tired and remote on return home.

The social life of the middle class young person in the teens outside the family was very limited. They were expected to go on family outings to visit family or friends. A minority of boys belonged to one of the new youth organizations such as the Boy Scouts. Group activities outside school with others of the same age were discouraged as likely to lead to trouble. Even with older teenagers, friendships with the opposite sex were closely watched and regulated with fathers taking responsibility for deciding on the time, usually 9.30 or 10 pm when the young person would be expected home.

2.6 **The life of the working class young in their teen years 1914–1960**

The outbreak of the First World War in 1914 followed a period of unparalleled chauvinism in political life and in the British press. Public schools had been hotbeds of patriotism for many years, preaching the imperial ethic of duty and the need to defend British interests with military strength. The hierarchy in these schools and the expectation of obedience and conformity made ideal military material. Schools right down the social scale were equally imbued with patriotism. For several years before 1914, as a result of war fever pumped up by the tabloid media, war with Germany had appeared inevitable and indeed, in some quarters, highly desirable.

For the first two years of the war, voluntary enlistment was sufficient to meet military needs. But by 1916, those needs had become much greater and the enthusiasm of the young to volunteer had been vastly diminished by the size of the casualty lists. Compulsory conscription from the age of 18 up to 35 was introduced in that year, and the eighteenth birthday suddenly became an entry ticket to a lottery in which the winning tickets won survival, but severe incapacity or death were to be the fate of many. Some young men looked forward to the time when they would be regarded as mature enough to enter the army, but many did not and certainly most of their parents did not. While for the middle classes the age of eighteen was already a dividing line between adolescence and adulthood, this had not been the case for working class young people. Now, with enthusiasm for the war at a low ebb, working class parents did not want their children to go to the trenches. They too began to see the period of life from 14 to 18 years as deserving special protection.

Eighteen years had not always been seen as the lower age limit when it was appropriate for young people to engage in military service. The Navy had always previously taken ordinary seamen and midshipmen much younger than this and expected boys in their teen years to play their part in combat. In the American Civil War, although both the Union and Confederate sides introduced compulsory conscription from the age of 18 years in 1862, it was common for younger males to fight. Indeed, in 1864, a strong battalion of 200 cadets all aged 15–17 years from the Virginia Military Institute charged and helped to put Union forces to flight at the battle of New Market in the Shenandoah Valley. No one saw anything wrong with this and indeed the heroism of the cadets is still celebrated in the South. So the First World War was an important landmark in the development of the view that young people under 18 years required shielding from some, at least, of the rigours of adult life.

Between the First and Second World War, there was hardly any time for this attitude to dissipate. There were only 15 years between 1918 when the first war ended and 1933 when Hitler came to power and the second war threatened. Compulsory National Service was introduced after the Second World War ended in 1945 and remained in force until 1960, with most young men serving 18 months or 2 years once they had reached their eighteenth birthday. This birthday therefore remained a watershed marking the end of a phase of life for the whole youth population from 1916 to 1960. For middle class children the gradual lengthening of education made 18 years a fairly natural transition point, but for working class children this was not the case. Many in the working class continued to leave school at 14 years or, after 1945, at 15 years, but felt it was not worth settling down in employment before they reached 18 years, so they took temporary jobs to 'fill in'. The period from 14 or 15–18 years was therefore an unsettled time. So the two world wars and National Service helped to establish 18 years for the first time as the end of a phase of life for working class young people.

Life in other respects did not change all that much for young working class people in their teen years between 1914 and the 1950s. The small rise in the compulsory school leaving age meant that more time was spent in school, but for many the last couple of years were regarded as a waste of time, especially if there was a job waiting and they had achieved basic literacy and numeracy. Class sizes were large and schools in working class districts were generally poorly provided with facilities.

As far as social life was concerned, the music halls gradually faded out, but were replaced by the increasingly popular cinema. There were now cheap Saturday morning performances for the younger end of the age group, but cinema attendance spread throughout the week. Most working class young people could afford to go at least once a week. Congregating outside the cinema before and after a performance was a common way to meet friends and make new acquaintances. But groups of young men and women met in the streets outside their homes at other times and, for many, this was what going out for the evening really meant, gossiping with friends, flirting or, for boys, playing street football or cricket.

For most of this period, though wages were low, employment possibilities for young people were reasonably good. During the Depression from the late 1920s to the mid-30s, there was very serious unemployment in the north and west of England, Wales, and Scotland, with very considerable hardship, but the south and east remained reasonably prosperous. Most factories and businesses now allowed their employees two weeks holiday a year in the summer, and often this meant the whole family could go away to the English seaside to stay in a boarding house or small hotel. Right up to the end of their teenage years young people would usually accompany other members of the family on such holidays. They were attached to their families and usually lived with them, sometimes willingly and affectionately, sometimes not, until their twenties when they made stable, intimate relationships and married.

2.7 **Teenagers: transformation by the market 1960–1997**

Between the end of the Second World War in 1945 and the end of the 1950s, somewhat earlier for the working class and a bit later for the middle class, the market woke up to the spending power of young people in their mid to late teens and early twenties. Working class youngsters, starting to earn good money at the age of fifteen, though still living at home, were not giving more than a fraction of their earnings to their parents, who themselves were in work and earning reasonably well. Mark Abrams carried out a study for the London Press Exchange in the early 1960s and identified the 'affluent teenager' as a powerful consumer. Of course, not all teenagers were affluent. Some were unemployed and others were on very low wages. In the middle class, the affluence of teenagers depended largely on how much pocket money they were given by their parents and this, in turn, depended on how much surplus their parents had available. There were many middle class parents on low pay. All the same, there were quite sufficient affluent teenagers to make marketing to them worthwhile.

As we have seen, the term 'teenager' was first coined in the 1940s in the United States, promoted into everyday language from the world of advertising and marketing. Young people in American high schools were thought to be readily identifiable, open to new products, and easy to sell to. The term crossed the Atlantic, but in Britain the world of austerity following the war was not immediately conducive to such focused marketing. By the late 1950s that situation had changed.

Marketing to an age group does not usually transform it. The successful merchandising of clothes to be worn in pregnancy, prams and baby clothes by MotherCare did not transform the process of reproduction. Saga has not transformed retirement or old age. Marketing to 13–18-year-olds did create a new brand of young person and acted as a transforming catalyst to the image of this age group. It turned teenagers into eager consumers of products specially fashioned for them and unsuitable both for children and young adults. It encouraged them to seek status and pleasure by demonstrating their awareness of the latest fashion in music and clothes. It legitimated their wish to demonstrate sexual attractiveness. By encouraging the teenage population to make up its own mind about what it wanted, focused marketing tackled adolescent ambivalence about separation from the family by strongly supporting its wish for independence and discouraging dependency. It created a very specific generational, relatively classless awareness. Gradually, middle class teenagers embraced the teenage culture. The culture they adopted was the same as the working class had already adopted. The social class convergence of taste among young people in the 1960s and the 70s was unprecedented.

2.8 Teenagers: transformation of social life 1960–1997

But the lives of teenagers did not change solely because of the marketing directed towards them. There were also important changes in the adult world, especially the world of young adults, brought about by economic affluence, the feminist movement, the contraceptive pill, and the media that changed the lives of teenagers more indirectly. Sexual freedom, empowered by the availability of the contraceptive pill, percolated down to teenagers from the world of young unmarried adults. There was greater convergence between the sexes. Girls became more overtly sexual in their behaviour. Boys and girls enjoyed the same sorts of music. The 1960s teenage pop culture was universally embraced. Academically girls started to study the same subjects as boys, began to catch up, and in the end did catch up and overtake boys in examination results even in mathematics and the sciences.

It gradually became the norm for both boys and girls to have had full sexual intercourse by the age of 16–17 years. Greater sexual freedom was but one reflection of the hedonism of the 1960s and its rejection of the puritan work ethic. Consumption of alcohol increased and continued to increase through the 1970s to the 90s in the young adult population and then among teenagers. Using illegal drugs, especially cannabis and then, in the 1990s, ecstasy, similarly increased both in young adults and in teenagers. There were changed attitudes to fidelity in marriage. Many more teenagers, around one in four, lived through the separation, divorce, and often remarriage of their parents, and many who did not have this experience saw their friends go through it. Cohabitation, though it did not replace marriage, became more popular. Though often relatively stable, it proved less durable than legal marriage. This meant both that increasingly teenagers entered into cohabiting relationships and more teenagers had parents who were cohabiting rather than married.

These changes in family life brought inevitable strain. Parents who had been brought up very differently found it hard to accept the freedom their teenage children wanted. The emotions experienced by both parents and teenagers were often so intense, it was impossible to communicate them adequately.

The step-parenting of adolescents proved to be a particularly tough task, as tough as being an adolescent stepchild. Attempted suicide became a common way for teenagers, especially teenage girls, to express their despair at their inability to persuade their parents or their boyfriends how they felt.

In the late 1970s and 80s, economic recession changed the lives of teenagers in other ways. Teenage boys living in manufacturing areas suddenly saw the employment opportunities they had taken for granted disappear within half a decade. Unemployment soared, especially in the north of England and Scotland and especially in the young. Indeed, youth unemployment extended into inner cities throughout the country. This had the effect of excluding many young people from the consumption of fashionable clothes and music that were so much part of the teenage lifestyle. The deprived and disadvantaged areas affected by the recession then saw an increase in signs of disaffection in the teenage population. An increase in violent behaviour on the streets, in disruptive behaviour in schools, in running away from home all occurred in the 1980s, but was largely confined to these poor areas of the country.

The government response to the recurrence of the 'youth problem' was to create training schemes. Youth Opportunities Schemes and Youth Training Programmes were introduced for early school leavers. These schemes were relatively unsuccessful, but had the effect of increasing the dependency of working class young people into the late teens, thus mimicking the social situation of the young middle class. However by this time, a much higher proportion of middle class youth were entering higher education and remaining dependent on their parents at least until their early and often to their mid-twenties. Also by this time the distinction between the lifestyle of those in their teen years and young adults had virtually disappeared. So-called 'post-modern' youth, hedonistic, avoiding committed relationships, but enjoying a range of experiences in different relationships, sometimes living with their parents and sometimes away from home, extended from 15 or 16 years to the mid-twenties. The teenage brand had disappeared, once again absorbed into a much longer period of 'youth' very much as had been the case right up to the mid-nineteenth century. The boundaries of the teenage years now dissolved both at the beginning with the appearance of 'tweenies' and at the end when so-called 'emergent adulthood' arrived.

Despite all these apparent dramatic changes, there were many ways in which the lives of young people in their teenage years in the decades following the Second World War were not all that different from the lives of those who went through their teens before it. The great majority of young people of this age lived with their parents throughout their teens and remained on reasonably good terms with them. Their values and attitudes remained remarkably similar to those of their parents. For most, attending school and achieving reasonable academic attainments remained important. For girls, friendships and conversation remained high among the pleasures of life, as did competitive games among boys. The teenage lifestyle came and then disappeared, but the fact remains that many boys and girls in the 1990s were, in many important ways, living much the same lives as their predecessors in the fifties.

Further, the fact that the values and attitudes of those in their teens in different social classes coalesced did not mean that class inequalities were abolished. Far from it, particularly in the UK and the USA (less in most other westernized countries), the income disparities between rich and poor families containing a young person in the teens have widened considerably. In a society where values are greatly influenced by material possessions and where the identity of the young is largely formed by the clothes they wear, the music they can afford to buy, the clubs they can afford to go to, disparities of income often lead to envy and frustration among young people of this age living in poverty.

2.9 The creation of diversity in the lives of the teens

All these changes in the lives of young people in their teens meant the creation of much greater variation in the lives they led. Before 1960, about nine out of ten 16-year-olds were living with both their biological parents. By the 1990s, this was only true for about 7 out of 10. In 1960, only about one in ten young people went to University. By the end of the twentieth century, the figure was approaching 50%. Before 1960, only a small number of 16–17-year-olds had had full sexual intercourse, but by the 1990s around half of them had had this experience. Before 1960, hardly any young people used illegal drugs. Now half the 16-year-old population has at least experimented with such drugs and many use them regularly. Leisure activities too have diversified. Videos and computer games have come on the market and now take up a good deal of the time of half the teenage population. So, as the examples at the beginning of Chapter 1 illustrate, family life, relationships, and leisure activities have changed in such a way that the lives of those in their teen years is immensely more variable than it used to be.

2.10 Adolescence in traditional societies

The evidence (from historical studies) that the teen years can be more or less happily lived in many different ways is given support by studies of traditional societies. The first and most famous of these was reported in 1928 by the anthropologist, Margaret Mead, in her book 'Coming of Age in Samoa'.

She proposed that personality in adolescents was closely linked to the sort of upbringing they had. In Samoa, she claimed, a relaxed, permissive upbringing, with children and those in their teens spreading their affection among many adults, a form of diffuse authority in large families with many adults in charge, early sexual knowledge, and the freedom to experiment all resulted in Samoan girls, with few exceptions, having a 'perfect adjustment'.

Margaret Mead's work has been seriously challenged, but, as with many pioneers, although much of what she wrote has now been discredited because it was based on accounts the young made up to please her, she stimulated an interest in the ways in which adolescents live their lives in different cultures throughout the world. Since her time, vast numbers of studies of adolescence in traditional societies have been carried out.

These have been most helpfully brought together by Alice Schlegel and Herbert Barry. They looked at information mainly collected by other anthropologists and psychologists from 186 pre-industrial societies. They range alphabetically from the Abipon, nomadic raiders on horseback of Spanish settlers in northern Argentina, through the Kung Bushmen of South West Africa, small nomadic independent groups, technologically primitive, primarily gatherers and secondarily hunters, to the Zuni of central western Mexico, primarily cultivating cereal grains, but secondarily engaged in husbandry of sheep and goats. What emerges from their findings is the tremendous diversity and variation of teen life in these societies. There is, it appears, no human group in which there is no gap between reaching physical sexual maturity and having full adult responsibilities. Schlegel and Barry therefore refer to 'the necessity of adolescence', but the gap may be and indeed often is as short as a year for girls and no more than two or three years for boys.

Most (around three quarters) of the societies studied had rituals or initiation rites round about the time that young people completed the physical changes of puberty. But this means that around one-quarter did not have such rituals. Further, although Schlegel and Barry refer to these as initiation rites marking the start of adolescence, as less than half the societies in which this was studied had a separate word for adolescence, in fact, in many of these societies, the rites marked an entry into young adulthood. In nearly all the societies, following the rituals, young people were expected to carry out new roles in, for example, employment, religious ceremonies, or military service. What is striking is the degree to which the young people were widely seen as useful, contributing to the community in many different ways. Here there was rather little diversity.

Variety was again apparent in sexual behaviour in those in their teens. For example, sexual intercourse was permitted, even encouraged in just under a third of these traditional societies, but forbidden in the remainder. There was therefore an enormous range of attitudes to premarital sex, ranging from the most permissive in the Polynesian islands to many societies in the Middle East in which a girl was often killed if she lost her virginity before marriage whether she had consented to sex or not.

The notion of the inevitability of conflict between young people in their teens and their parents is also refuted by anthropological studies. On a 10-point scale in which moderate conflict was rated 5, and severe conflict was rated 8, the average score for boys' conflict with their fathers was 3.7 and with their mothers was 2.7. For girls the conflict score was 2.8 with both fathers and mothers. In contrast, the mean scores for 'intimacy' or emotional closeness with both parents were much higher, ranging from 4.1 to 7.2. Though there was much diversity, it seems as though in traditional societies relations between those in their teens and their parents are marked more by affection than by serious discord.

Finally what is striking about these traditional societies is the way the people who live in them think of the different phases of life; what marks one phase off from another is not chronological age as much as marriage or parenthood. So in societies in which marriage is relatively late, occurring in the twenties, those in their teens are grouped with those in their early and mid-twenties and called youths or young adults.

The contrast between western concepts of adolescence and those of other cultures is strikingly seen in immigrant families. Sami Timimi, in discussing the adolescence of immigrant Arab families has pointed especially to the much greater importance given in such families to the social construction of the self. In the West adolescence is seen as a time of greatly increasing autonomy and individuation. Arab families, in contrast, value greater affiliation to the family. The bond between mother and child is lifelong and unseverable. Indeed in rural Arab settings, adolescence has little importance as a life stage, and is unmarked by any ritual or ceremony. Parents are expected to find work for their children as well as a suitable marriage partner.

2.11 **The social construction of adolescence**

In some societies such as our own, the needs of the adult world change from time to time. Then the adult world changes its mind about the sort of adolescents it needs. This too has been studied, though less intensively. For example, in 1972 Klaus Riegel, a social psychologist working in the United States, suggested that modern psychologic theories, just like those current in the Middle Ages, about the way young people behaved, emerged from the dominant political and economical ideologies. They were not developed in a social vacuum. Riegel wrote that it was 'naïve, irrelevant and irresponsible to anchor our scientific efforts upon an abstract truth criterion traditionally conceived as either "god-given" or as provided by the "scientific facts" and "nature" itself'. The 'truths' that psychologists discovered, he suggested, depended on the values held by the societies in which they lived and worked. What was 'true' in one society would not hold in another.

Robert Enright and his colleagues from the Department of Educational Psychology in the University of Wisconsin carried out a study to test Riegel's theory with respect to adolescence. They looked at the way economic conditions and whether the country was at war affected the views of American psychologists about the nature of adolescence. Enright examined all the articles published in the *Journal of Genetic Psychology*, the only psychological journal published continuously since the late nineteenth century. They analyzed all the articles concerning the entire age spectrum traditionally associated with adolescence. They then compared the terms used about adolescents in four different time periods: a period of economic depression between 1894 and 1898; the time of American involvement in World War I from 1917 to 1918; the period of the Great Depression between 1933 and 1936; and the period of American involvement in World War II from 1943 to 1945. Three independent judges examined 89 articles in all, roughly equally divided between these four periods.

The judges were asked to look for the terms used to describe adolescents and for the assumptions that psychologists made about them. Were they regarded as childlike? For example, one article described them as showing 'the same restlessness and irregularity in application to their task that one sees in very young children'. Or were they thought of as more like adults? One psychologist advocated 'citizen soldiers' and 'juvenile employment' for adolescents. Was adolescence a fast developmental stage, with rapid transition to adulthood? A well-known psychologist called Merrill wrote that adolescents by age 16 were 'mature enough … to take care of themselves under all conditions, strong enough to stand the rigors of hard work on the farm'. Should education accelerate the adolescent stage? G. Stanley Hall himself in 1918 referred to the American adolescent as 'callow, shambling … boys are growing wild and slightly criminal'. He praised some high schools for having 'real rifle practice like military manoeuvres'.

What Enright found was that during World War I, psychologists consistently portrayed adolescents as more grown-up and mature than those who had written in the earlier economic depression. During wartime they saw adolescence as a more rapid period of psychological growth than during the economic depression. Generally young people in economic depressions were seen as more childlike than in wartime. Enright concluded 'when youth are not needed in the work force, theorists paint a childlike picture of teenagers. When youth are needed to tend victory gardens, to work in factories, or to fight in battle, theorists more frequently paint a more rugged, adult-like portrait of youth'.

The same is true today. In the late 1990s and at the beginning of the twenty-first century, young men in their mid-teens have been described as heroes if they are manfully fighting for the 'right' side, but immature, weak, and misguided if taking part in combat for terrorist groups we deplore. During the civil war in Kosovo in 1999, when their fathers had been taken away and killed, brave 13-year-old Albanian boys were described approvingly when they took up arms or drove tractors carrying the family possessions to safety. Mohammed Humay, a 15-year-old Afghan boy whose chieftain father was killed, commanded 300 soldiers of the Northern Alliance, and was seen as a much-admired 'warlord' in the western press, while Serbian and Taliban 16- and 17-year-olds taking part in combat in the Balkans in the late 1990s and in Afghanistan in 2001 were viewed as misguided children.

Nowadays most young people in their teens are living in families, financially dependent on their parents well into their late teens. They are studying in schools where they have to conform to rules laid down 'for their own good' and then go on to universities where they have no responsibilities except to themselves until their early twenties. They are discouraged from forming stable relationships because society does not think they are ready for them. So in these circumstances, it is to be expected that the stereotype of the immature, moody, vulnerable adolescent, prone to violent aggression, sexually promiscuous, irresponsible, and incapable of taking responsibility, described in Chapter 1 should prevail. Hopefully, we are entering a period of greater awareness of the degree to which we 'invent' the sort of teenagers we need. A relatively new approach to understanding the way this happens has been pioneered by Alison Jones, Alan Prout, and a group of British sociologists, largely focusing on children, but sometimes also turning their attention to those in their teen years.

2.12 A footnote on 'adolescence' in the animal world

Can we find evidence for a separate phase of life between the onset of puberty and full adult status in the animal world? In fact, like humans in both traditional and western societies primates show an enormous variation in this respect. Patrice Huerre and his colleagues have reviewed the fascinating evidence, especially in lemurs, but also in baboons, chimpanzees, orangutans, and gorillas. They conclude that the life of juveniles varies not only from one species to another, but even within species depending on ecological conditions (especially the abundance or scarcity of food supplies), the geographical zone, and local demographic features. As in humans, the roles assigned to the young largely depend on the interests of the mature adult population.

Chapter 3

Teens in the family

3.1 **Introduction**

In Chapter 1, I suggested that most young people in their teens did not conform to the stereotypes the media and sometimes even professionals put out about them. In this chapter, I shall first look at the ways in which most of those in their teens actually do behave in families. Then I shall go on to suggest that one of the most important reasons why most teenage children do not show the appalling behaviour their reputation might lead one to expect is that their parents have, since early childhood, taken account of their children's feelings, listened to them, and eventually arrived at family relationships that are reasonably democratic. They have empowered their children.

In the first chapter, I detailed some of the myths about the behaviour and moods of those in their teen years. One of these suggests that young people, as they reach puberty, start to engage in serious ill-tempered confrontations with their parents. Such constant arguments, it is said, are necessary for normal development in adolescence. They persist throughout the teens. Without them, the adolescent cannot achieve the independence necessary to be a mature adult. How accurate is this picture?

Alan is a 25-year-old teacher. His parents are in their late fifties. When asked what he was like as a child, they describe him as having always been easy to manage. It was no trouble getting him to eat or off to sleep. He found it a little difficult to settle at infant school, but after that he always attended school regularly and, though he found some lessons difficult, especially maths, he always tried hard and eventually achieved good enough results to train to be a teacher. During his teen years, his mother used to joke about the fact that he wasn't a normal teenager because he always kept to the rules his parents laid down. He linked up with a group of boys he went out with from primary school, none of whom were ever in trouble and he still sees two or three of these. His only significant conflicts in the teen years were with his older sister, with whom he became rather possessive when she began to go out with boys. He himself began to have girlfriends at around 16 years and eventually formed a steady relationship with a school secretary, a young woman a year older than himself whom he met at his work. They are now living together and plan to marry. Alan sees his parents once a week at weekends, and is in phone contact at some other time during the week. He still finds talking to his parents helpful when thinking about big life decisions, such as changing his job or buying a flat. He is fond of them as they are of him.

Helen, Alan's girlfriend, is a 26-year-old school secretary. Her parents separated when she was only two years old and she and her mother were alone together for three years before her mother met another man and shortly afterwards, married him. She hasn't seen her first father since the day he left. Helen was always slightly resentful of her stepfather from the time he entered her family. His arrival coincided with her starting infant school and she showed a good deal of clinging behaviour for the first term before she settled down. However, her stepfather took care not to intrude on the relationship between his wife and stepdaughter. He encouraged them to spend time together. When Helen was 14 years old she started to go out with boys. Her stepfather thought this was too young, but he kept his views to himself and let his wife deal with the hassles and arguments that arose over times she was expected back in the evenings, the mess in her room, and the four or five times she came home drunk. Helen and her mother were very close (too close thought some of her friends!), and when she met Alan she was twenty three and still living at home. She also sees her mother and stepfather once a week and phones her mother in-between times. She remains emotionally distant from her stepfather. He regrets this as he always has, but he continues to have a loving relationship with his wife and accepts the limits of his stepdaughter's love. Helen and Alan get on well. He is very confident of her love for him and she a little less so of his. She checks up on him when he is out and she does not know where he is. He does not like this but accepts that this is part of her nature.

3.2 **Three out of four trouble-free teens**

The stories of Alan and Helen are unremarkable. They have both had a relatively smooth time from when they were young children right up to their mid-twenties. From reading the textbooks and sometimes from reading self-help books for parents of teenagers, one might think there is something deeply wrong with them. Where is the anger? Where is the protest? What has happened to all that normal emotional turmoil that marks the adolescent period? Surely the blandness of their existence must mean they have missed out on life. Well, they may have missed out on some aspects of the excitement that can form part of being young. But the fact is that evidence from a number of surveys strongly suggests that around three out of four people reach and go through their teen years and early adulthood in a rather similar way to the two individuals I have described. Of course that still leaves one in four.

In other chapters and later in this one, I shall describe far more troubled and troublesome individuals. But when Helen and Alan see such children and young people, as they do at the school where they both work, they are far from envious. They feel they were the lucky ones. They are perhaps not aware of the importance of their own stable and optimistic temperaments to the smoothness of their early lives. They do recognize the benefits they had in the love and security their parents gave them, as well as the opportunity they both had to have their say and express their feelings when there was the possibility of conflict between them and their parents.

They are not at all untypical. In a survey carried out in 2002 by the Future Foundation in which 500 13- to 18-year-olds were interviewed, 85% agreed with the statement 'I'm happy with my family life'. Only one in ten said they definitely did not get on with their parents. One in three had not argued with their parents during the last 12 months.

3.3 **The troubled or troublesome one in four**

The fact that three out of four young people go through their teens in reasonable tranquillity, means that quite a number do not. Most of the rest are not showing deep disturbance either, but around one in four of the total, for at least part of their teen years, either experience significant inner distress or make life very difficult for those around them. As seen in Chapter 2, some authorities would regard these as going through adolescence 'normally' and the distress they experience or the trouble they cause as part of 'normal' adolescence. Whatever one's view about this, it is clear that this is not a happy time for many in their teens. Further, some of these troubled young people were not troubled in their earlier childhood and will live more tranquil lives when they reach their twenties.

Among the one in four there is a small number who are really disturbed and in need of help. The great majority of these have problems described in other chapters. They include extreme forms of depression, anxiety, anorexia, drug and alcohol problems, aggressive behaviour, or a mixture of these.

But let us pause for a moment and think whether this makes the teens a 'special' time of life. All the evidence suggests that at every phase of life, whether it is in childhood or in adult life, around three in five are free of upset, most of the remainder have relatively minor but unpleasant inner experiences, and a small proportion are really very disturbed. The teens are like every other time of life in this respect.

There is another way in which those in their teens are similar to people at other ages. Some young people in their teens who show a degree of upset have had similar experiences or shown similar behaviour in childhood and many of these will continue to show such problems in their twenties and beyond. This is especially the case for the more troubled among them. This is exactly what one finds at other ages—a minority who are showing problems that have existed for some time and will persist into the future, and another, larger group showing temporary, more short-lived upset.

3.4 **The family as the cradle of tranquillity or disaffection**

In other chapters, I shall discuss the ways in which the tranquil majority pass through their teens coping positively with the challenges it presents. I then go on to discuss those less fortunate. In each case, whether one is considering upsets of mood, difficulties of behaviour, sexual life, drugs and alcohol, nutrition, or self-confidence about appearance, the cradle of tranquillity or of disaffection is the family. When particular difficulties occur, there are always special reasons why it is these and not others that surface, but the way the family members get on with each other and communicate is always important.

Families do not live in a vacuum. They exist in a social world that may make things easier or much, much more difficult for them. Living with teens in areas with high rates of poverty and unemployment, poor inner-city schools, and a lack of leisure facilities is a very different experience from living in a leafy suburb where your next door neighbour has a swimming pool. Other social influences affect all families, no matter what their income level. The media, for example, affect all families, no matter what their social level.

Just as social conditions vary, making it much easier for some parents to bring up their children, so children themselves vary. As Judith Rich Harris has pointed out, they are not all made out of the same building materials. I shall discuss in more detail later in this chapter the importance of the child's temperament in deciding just how parents behave towards their children.

So although in what follows I have put emphasis on the way parents bring up their children, this should not be read as meaning parents are to blame when things go wrong. In my experience, all parents do their best for their children. But some have a much, much harder task than others, because of the stressed circumstances in which they live, because of their own mental health problems, especially anxiety, depression, and drug misuse, or because their children have inherited difficult temperaments.

In what follows in this chapter, I shall first consider what we know about the way relationships develop in families that make it more or less likely that those in their teens will enjoy a relatively smooth and enjoyable experience.

Then I shall discuss how policy makers who influence the sort of society we live in might make it easier for parents and their teen children to achieve this result.

3.5 Types of parenting

In the 1960s, Diana Baumrind, an American psychologist, described different ways parents behaved to their children before, during, and after puberty. Although her ideas have since been questioned, they have largely stood the test of time. There were, Baumrind said, two different and contrasting approaches to the upbringing and especially the disciplining of children and adolescents—authoritarian and authoritative. Neglectful or indifferent parents who, for one reason or another, find it impossible or unnecessary to provide care and supervision form another group.

Authoritarian parents put emphasis on obedience and conformity. They do not consult or negotiate with their children over decisions, being more likely just to give their decision in a non-negotiable fashion and shout or scream if their children make any attempt to argue with them. Their children are not rewarded for good behaviour and they prefer disciplinary methods that involve punishment, such as withdrawal of privileges, and gating or grounding.

Although other factors are also important, authoritarian and indifferent parents are much more likely to have adolescent children in trouble with the law. Their children are more often depressed and miserable, and more often take drugs and drink alcohol to a problematic extent. They do not do so well at school. Such findings sound as if they might lead to parent blaming, a tendency psychologists and teachers find difficult to avoid. So it is important to stress that authoritarian and indifferent parents have themselves had different sorts of upbringing. In addition, their children have often been temperamentally difficult from the start, and may have elicited stricter behaviour from them. As far as their own childhoods are concerned, they have much more often been beaten for disobedience in childhood, and have not been listened to themselves. They are also more likely to be living in difficult circumstances, under emotional stress, and with money worries of their own. Many parents who are seen as persecutors of their children have been victims of their own parents and are often currently victims of stress in their own lives.

3.6 Teenager abuse: a forgotten form of ill-treatment

ChildLine is a UK telephone helpline for children who are in distress and wish to talk to someone confidentially and anonymously about it. It receives around 130 000 calls a year of which about two-thirds are made by children aged 12 years and above. Of these about one in five are reporting physical and sexual abuse, and of these, nine out of ten say they have been abused by people they know, largely members of their own families. We know these figures only represent a fraction of those who are maltreated. In the US, it is reckoned that about one in three of recognized cases of abuse are of young people in their teens. In the UK, official figures suggest a lower proportion, but it is still sizeable.

The pattern of abuse in the teens is different from that in younger children. Sexual abuse is more common, and, though a higher proportion of stepfathers than biological fathers abuse their children, because there are so many more biological fathers, more abuse overall is committed by biological fathers. Physical abuse usually involves excessive physical punishment by mothers and not, again as is commonly thought, by stepfathers. An American study of abuse of adolescents carried out in the mid-1980s found nearly three in five were abused by their birth mothers, one in three by their birth fathers, and only one in twenty-five by a stepfather or mother's boyfriend. As the number of stepfamilies has increased, probably the numbers of stepfathers is greater now, but it is still much smaller than commonly believed.

Abuse may take many forms. The child may be rejected, terrorized, ignored, isolated, or corrupted, for example, by sexual seduction, or by initiation into inappropriate use of drugs and alcohol. The impact of abuse on the young person may involve running away, followed by prostitution and a high risk of contracting an HIV infection.

Cases of abuse of young children frequently hit the headlines. Indeed, victims such as Maria Colwell and Victoria Climbié sometimes become almost household names. Those in their teens are much less often given publicity, yet the frequency of abuse within the family of young people of this age is little less than that of children. If one includes abuse outside the family, such as in school, then abuse is more common in the teens than it is in earlier years. So why is it so often ignored?

One reason is that, as far as teenaged children are concerned, far more publicity is given to the results of abuse than to its causes. Much attention is given to the very large numbers of runaways in their teens. These are exposed to other high-profile types of disadvantage, such as homelessness, running away, prostitution, and drug use. But these are most frequently consequences of ill-treatment in the family. Of course, runaways need attention, but it is important to look at the reasons behind their wish to leave their families even if that means living in squalor.

The abuse of adolescents within families requires many explanations. One almost invariable finding is the presence of particular types of parenting.

It is well established that children who have been brought up using authoritarian or over-permissive, neglectful methods are much more likely to be abused than are those who have been brought up in authoritative families. Parents who consult with their children and who listen to their views before making decisions are much, much less likely to abuse them.

Charlie was 17 years old when he was picked up by the police sleeping roughly near Kings Cross Station in London. He had never before told his story to anyone in authority. His father was a security guard, brought up himself by an army sergeant who had instilled in him the need for strict discipline from an early age. Charlie's father had been frequently beaten for misdemeanours, and he followed this example with his own son. He frequently beat him for misbehaviour from about the age of 2 years. At the beginning he was punished in this way for not eating all his lunch or messing himself when he did not get to the lavatory in time. His mother was entirely under the control of her dominating, bullying husband. As a 12-year-old, Charlie was beaten for not keeping his room clean and tidy. However, by the time he was 14 years old he was the same size as his father and began to hit back. There were fierce physical fights. Eventually, Charlie also hit his mother whom he felt had failed to protect him, walked out of the house, and caught the train from the Midlands town where he lived, for London. He had no educational qualifications sufficient to get him a job. Fortunately, he was picked up by the police before he was involved in prostituting himself, a likely outcome otherwise.

When Charlie's parents were contacted, they gave a different story. They said they could not have him home again. He had always been a difficult child. Recently he had been violent to both of them on several occasions, and they saw him as out of their control. Charlie's father agreed he had been a strict father, but saw the beatings he had given as fully deserved. He himself had been treated like that and it had done him no harm. Indeed he felt severe punishment had helped him to tell the difference between right and wrong and his strict discipline was intended to benefit his son, not to harm him.

This story, very typical for young people picked up on the street in London and other big cities, illustrates the way harsh parenting can result in parents getting caught up in physical fights with their children. There are many reported examples of young people in their teens inflicting more harm on their parents than they have had inflicted on them, but the cycle of violence nearly always starts with parents. Charlie's father is typical in seeing his own behaviour as enforcing discipline rather than abusing his son.

Occasionally, this sort of abuse actually starts in the teen years, usually as a result of a change in relationships at that time, but much more commonly, as was the case with Charlie, the pattern has been going on from earlier childhood.

Programmes for runaway teenagers, for drug addicts, for male and female young prostitutes operating in big cities are all necessary to deal with the casualties of harsh parenting. In a later section of this chapter, I shall discuss how such problems might be prevented from occurring in the first place. For the moment let us just note that abuse of adolescents is far more common than is generally realized. Further, the abuse of teenaged children is just an extreme of a form of parenting that arises because some parents think they have the right to treat their children of this age in any way they want.

3.7 Indulgent parenting

Diana Baumrind's work was elaborated by other psychologists who described other types of parenting with poor outcome—indulgent and indifferent or permissive. Indulgent parents are warm towards their children, but tend to be passive, accepting, and uninterested in setting standards for their children's learning or behaviour, while indifferent parents are neglectful and fail to supervise their children adequately. Often over-indulgent parents have had an unusually strict upbringing themselves, and are determined to avoid such behaviour towards their own children. They are quite unable to say 'no' to their children's demands. Not surprisingly this leads to their children running into severe difficulties in the outside world, when they assume they are going to have their own way there as they do with their parents.

As with physical abuse, neglect and over-indulgence are usually seen as forms of behaviour shown by parents to young children. But they are equally damaging to those in their teens.

3.8 Authoritative parents

In contrast to authoritarian parents, *authoritative* parents do listen and negotiate, and are prepared to make reasonable compromises, though they stick firmly to boundaries once they think they have gone as far as they can. They tend to give children more responsibility and, in return, expect and get more help in the house. Their children take greater responsibility and do more regular jobs around the house. Throughout childhood and the teen years, they change their rules and expectations as their children become more competent, mature, and responsible.

Parents who bring up their children this way, not surprisingly, have a warmer, closer, and more affectionate relationship with them when they are of teen age. Their children have a low risk of delinquency. They are less often depressed, drink less alcohol, are less involved with illegal drug taking. They do better at school. They are more caring to others. Young student activists determined to reduce inequality and injustice in the world and to preserve the environment are likely to have been brought up by authoritative parents.

It has sometimes been suggested that authoritative parenting may be a great idea for middle class families in north America, Europe, and Australasia, but is quite inappropriate in working class families and in other societies with different social structures. Now obviously, family structure and function vary greatly from culture to culture, but the benefits of authoritative parenting seem widespread. Since Baumrind published her findings 40 years ago, studies in different social groups in the United States, in East and West Germany before the unification of the country, and in other parts of the world, have all confirmed her findings. Authoritative is best everywhere!

So what are the essential ingredients of authoritative parenting? Parents who listen to and consult with their teenage children just have to be interested in them as individuals. In the jargon, they have to be child-centred. In all probability, as we shall see later in this chapter, they will have been child-centred since their children were born. They will have observed and taken note of their children's ways of showing distress and pleasure, even if these are subtle and difficult for other people to confirm. They will respect their children's preferences for certain foods, clothing, and friends. They will adjust their level of supervision to the child's level of competence so their practices will change as the child gets older. They may well be very firm over some areas of disagreement, but much more relaxed over others. They will be firm when they need to be for the safety of the child, but they will let their children learn from their own mistakes when it is not dangerous to do so.

A reminder. All this emphasis on parenting ignores one very important element in the way parents 'bring up' their children, namely what children themselves bring to the manufacture of relationships within the family. As anyone who has been involved with groups of young children or has had more than one child of their own knows, children vary greatly, from a very early age, in their temperaments. Some are active and demanding, others passive and accepting. Some are amazingly compliant, others constantly testing the limits. Some take readily to new experiences, others take ages to warm up when they are in a new situation.

These differences affect the way parents treat their children. When parents say to me they treat all their children exactly the same, I express some doubt whether this is really possible. Of course, every parent tries to give children presents of the same value and to avoid having favourites, but children do not let you treat them the same. They make parents behave in different ways. Active, inquisitive, exploring children will make parents behave more firmly than passive, withdrawn children, whose parents will want to draw them out and let them experiment. *Children bring up their parents, just as parents bring up their children.* And, it must be admitted, some children bring up their parents well and others rather badly! It is very likely that authoritative parents have children who behave better when they are consulted and have, at least to some degree, shaped their parents' behaviour, as well as being shaped by it. Authoritative parents with children who tend to be chaotic and impulsive will provide firmer structure in their lives than those who have inhibited, anxious offspring.

3.9 **Numerous stresses upset family relationships**

Relationships between children and 'authoritative' parents are not always smooth. There are sometimes uncomfortable bumps in the road. When problems arise in relationships involving adolescents, this is usually put down to the 'nature of the beast'. Adolescents were always thus, is the cry. What can you expect? It's the hormones, the phase of life, the being in the in-between years. As seen in Chapter 1, these are weak and unsatisfactory explanations. It is very much more likely that difficulties in parent–teenage relationships have arisen because of circumstances that would be upsetting at any age, especially, as we shall also see in other chapters, in the clustering together of stresses.

At any phase of life, facing new experiences is anxiety provoking. The 5-year-old going to 'proper' school for the first time, the 20-year-old starting his first job, the 40-year-old having to make new relationships after a painful separation from a long-standing partner, the 60-year-old facing a life of retirement, the 80-year-old with a terminal illness, these are all people who will, at least if they are ordinary human beings, suffer anxiety because they are facing new experiences. Some people become rather withdrawn when they are anxious, others are irritable. Most young people in their teen years face more new experiences than they have done in the past or will do in the future. Their teen years are likely to present them with their first sexual experience, their first serious taste of alcohol, their first public examinations, their first opportunity to drive a car, the first occasion they are offered illegal drugs. They too will be anxious and they too may become withdrawn or irritable as a result. The harmony of family life, even with authoritative parents, may well be rocked when this occurs.

It is not just poor preparation that makes for serious disturbances. Poverty, overcrowded housing, lack of employment, an absence of affordable leisure facilities will all make it more likely that strain will occur. When people are already stressed to the limit to work out how to make ends meet, the fact that an adolescent in the family is finding it hard to cope with a new experience, will not have much impact. Communication between family members and the opportunity to use those valuable negotiating skills will be reduced in families living in poverty. It is well known that children in families living in poverty are under increased strain. Inevitably both parents and children will be less sensitive to each other's needs. The opportunities to use and develop emotional 'intelligence' (see Chapter 9) will be reduced.

3.10 Authoritative parenting begins at birth: the 'attachment' story

Much emphasis is now placed by psychologists on the importance of the development of an 'attachment' bond between parent and the young infant for healthy emotional development. Mothers and fathers begin to link up with their babies at birth. Within a few hours, the baby is starting to take an active part in this linking process. From then on these 'attachment' relationships are at the heart of the behaviour and emotional development of children first to their parents and, by the age of 2 or 3 years, to other people.

For successful attachment to occur, it is necessary for parents to be 'attuned' to the signals the infant puts out. From the first hours of life, mothers strive to recognize when their babies want to feed and when they have had enough. Later this need to be sensitive to the baby's needs will extend to striving to understand the reason why the baby is crying. Do they have a wet or soiled nappy? Are they tired? Do they want attention?

At the same time, it is clear that a baby can be more or less sensitive to the parent's moods and wishes. Long ago, psychoanalysts described the baby's capacity for 'primary empathy', or the instinctive capacity of the infant to 'read' and react to the mother's level of anxiety. It is now well established that babies change their behaviour, becoming restless and upset when a mother is depressed or even pretends to be depressed.

This mutual sensitivity to each other's needs and wishes makes it possible for mothers and babies to 'negotiate' with each other from the earliest days. The baby may be hungry, but the mother, whether she is breast or bottle feeding, may not feel for one reason or another that the time is right for another feed. Alternatively, the mother, her breasts heavy with milk or needing to get back to sleep, may want to feed while the baby may show little interest.

Somehow mother and baby have to sort these conflicting needs out and in doing so the basis of authoritative parenting is established. For parents, initially mainly the mother, need both to develop the capacity to be attuned to the young child's needs and to take responsibility for the decisions to be made. Successful parents discover what it is their babies want and negotiate with them, but this does not mean they always finish up giving in to them.

In the end it is parents who take the responsibility. The acceptance by the child of their parents' better judgement is the basis on which love, trust, and security are established. Emotionally healthy children therefore arrive at the teen years with a pattern of authoritative parenting already in place.

3.11 **Love thwarted, security threatened**

Difficulties in the early years of life may have made it difficult for this pattern to become established. The mother may have been depressed or preoccupied with financial problems or arguments with her partner so that she could not give her child the attention he needed for security and trust to be established. Alternatively, her baby or young child may not have been good at putting out readable signals. Towards the end of this chapter, I shall suggest various ways society can make it easier for parents and children to achieve strong positive attachments to each other. But if, for whatever reason, the child arrives at the teen years showing one or other of the patterns of insecure attachment that have been described, this will make authoritative parenting not impossible, but that much more difficult.

3.12 **Love and security in the teens as the basis for authoritative parenting**

Most young people arrive at their teen years with a strong positive attachment to their parents. They love them and feel secure in their parents love for them. Such attachment remains a basis for successful parenting throughout the teens and for healthy emotional development throughout life. During much of the twentieth century many psychological theories assumed it was healthy and desirable for children's attachment to their parents to diminish gradually throughout middle childhood and disappear altogether by adolescence. It was thought that it was thoroughly undesirable, if not dangerous, for close, warm attachments to parents to continue to exist when a child became sexually mature, for troubling incestuous desires would inevitably follow. Further, evolutionary theory dictated that young mature adults should be independent if they were to be successful. But then psychologists began to take notice of the fact that young people in their teen years mostly remained warm, friendly, and loving to their parents throughout this time and indeed into young adulthood and beyond. They began to study how young people in their teens showed attachment and in what ways this affected their behaviour and adjustment in other ways.

It rapidly became clear that the attachment between parents and their teenage children represented a most important and significant relationship on both sides. In general, and, of course this is not always the case, children in their teen years who are warm and affectionate to their parents, who like having their parents around a good bit of the time and confide in them and who, in return, are loved by their parents, show major advantages in other aspects of their lives. They see themselves as people better able to cope with difficulties. They have more friends and get on better with them than young people who are less attached or unattached to their parents. They show more caring behaviour to people who are upset and in need of sympathy. They are less likely to be depressed and anxious or to show behavioural difficulties. This is not to say that parents remain more important than friends as significant figures in a teenagers' lives. The reverse is usually the case. But it does mean that there are advantages to those teenagers who remain in good contact with their parents.

3.13 Continuity of attachment into adolescence and adult life

These findings strongly challenge the idea that the achievement of independence is prevented by having a warm, close relationship with one's parents. There is a good evidence to the contrary. Of course, the nature of attachment in adolescence is different from that in earlier childhood. The challenge for parents and young people themselves is to achieve separation in some respects, while continuing to connect in other ways. Psychologist Lindsay Chase-Lansdale and her colleagues have described the ideal end-product for the adolescent as 'the establishment of an identity that is separate from parents, a strong sense of autonomy, yet nested in the context of newly defined, more peer-like close emotional bonds with mother and father.' Put more simply, ideally children can gradually become adult friends of their parents. Such an outcome for adolescents sounds pretty good news for parents too. Naturally parents who are friends need to know when, like all other friends, they are not wanted around.

Those feelings that make up 'attachment' in young children are surely also those that make up the most important components of our close relationships with other people throughout the whole of our lives. They are found in girls and women who make friends in their early teens and remain friends for life, in our relationships with our parents in our own adult life, in young couples in romantic love, and in elderly married people who have been together for forty or more years. Less intensely, they are found throughout life in attachments made to colleagues at work and to less intimate friends with whom one shares common memories or interests in common. When these attachments are broken by separation or death, the pain is intense, as is the joy experienced when reunions occur after separation.

Attachment theorists would say that the first attachment of a baby to its mother is different because it programmes the baby for relationships later in life. Well, there is no doubt that a disastrous first parental attachment involving abuse or neglect is indeed very bad news for later life, though there are numerous examples to show it need not be irrecoverable. But so is being let down badly by a friend in one's teens or abused by a lover in one's thirties. Such experiences also reverberate into the future. So there is no good reason to downplay the importance of the attachments that remain, transformed though they may be, between teenage children and their parents.

3.14 **From authoritative parenting to family democracy**

Families where the parents are authoritative are not really 'democratic' in any absolute sense. In a democracy, it is assumed that everyone has an equally important vote. Clearly this cannot be the case for young children or even for those in their early teen years, but it can and does work in most aspects of life for parents and children in their mid- and late teenage years. Involving children in decision-making inevitably works differently at different ages. Two-year-olds in families where parents are 'attuned' to take into account their childrens' feelings, will help to make decisions. They may make clear how they would like to be put to bed, for example, by expressing their preferences for which doll or teddy they want to have with them in bed, how long they want the person who is tucking them up to stay with them, whether they want the light on or off, a drink by the bed, the door open or shut. These will all be matters for negotiation. There will not be very complicated discussions about them, but there will be negotiation. If parents are thinking of splitting up, there will not be negotiations with the two-year-old about whether they will separate or, if they do, whom she will live with or what the arrangements might be for visiting the other parent. But even very young children will make their feelings known about visiting arrangements and these may change as a result. Eight-year-olds in families whose parents are authoritative in their pattern of upbringing will be involved in decisions about many aspects of their own lives, their friends, and leisure activities, as well as decisions about family activities such as what to do at a weekend, what to eat for supper, what TV programmes to watch, or videos to borrow. They too would not be consulted about really major decisions concerning, for example, the separation of their parents, but they would be consulted about and much more deeply involved than two-year-olds in arrangements made after the separation. Up to and usually beyond this age, parents will have the final say on all decisions.

By the time the young reach their mid-teens, many families may have become democracies in a much more real sense, in which the child's view counts as much as the adult's. The range of decisions in which children are involved will have increased greatly. By this time, they will be much more frequently consulted on nearly all aspects of family life. Not only will they be consulted, but they will often have most say in the final decision. For example, when it comes to buying a new PC or a video, 15-year-olds are likely to have more information about the different features one should look out for than their parents.

In a study carried out early in the year 2000 by Abbey National of 950 British families, containing children aged from 8 to 15 years, in 65% the children helped to select the annual holiday destination, and 84% were involved in deciding weekend and leisure plans. Forty-two per cent involved their children in deciding whether to move house. Children in their teen years were, of course, involved more in making decisions than younger children. There has been a change over the last 30–40 years in the amount children are involved in decision-making. Around three quarters of mothers and fathers said that they involved their child in decision-making and communicated more with them than had been the case with their own parents.

The public relations firm that put out a summary of the Abbey National study headed its press release 'Pester Power is Good for Families'. The impression given was that children are only allowed into the decision-making process if they nag to be allowed to do so. This may well be the case in some families, but in democratic families parents realize not only that children should be involved because they are going to be affected by such decisions, but that their children may actually be the most informed members of the family. So they would be depriving themselves of useful expertise if they failed to involve their children.

As a toddler, Carla was a loving and lovable two-year-old most of the time, but extremely self-willed. She would shout and scream to get her own way. Bedtime was a nightmare as she tried to extend the time she was allowed to stay up. Her parents were driven to desperation at times, but they did not resort to smacking her. Instead they persisted in trying to make going to bed a more agreeable experience for her, telling her stories and giving in to her wishes for the light to be left on and for the door to be left open, but never letting her stay up longer than they felt was right. It took two years before she settled at night in less than 15 min. She reached puberty having had an otherwise settled earlier childhood. At 14 years, her parents hit problems again as they negotiated with her over the time that she was allowed to stay out at night with

*her first boyfriend. By finding rewards for a return home before 11 pm at week-
ends and earlier during the week, by continuing to show how much they cared
for her, and by avoiding gating except on one occasion, they managed to
persuade her mostly to return at a reasonable hour and were relieved that at least
she never stayed out all night. By this age she was taking part in all family
decisions concerning, for example, where to go on holiday and what computer
equipment to buy, though her parents took the final decisions. By 19 years,
when she was at College but living at home, Carla became fully involved in
discussions whether her father should retire from his job early. He was
unhappy there, but really needed to complete more years in order to qualify
for a reasonable pension. Carla's father did not take his daughter's view that he
might be better off being poor but happy, but it was an opinion he valued and
took into account. She had become a valued friend.*

3.15 **When caring is the other way round: young carers**

Traditionally, the early and mid-teen years are seen as a time when parents
continue to look after their children, gradually giving them more freedom, but
continuing to supervise their activities at least to some degree. Caring is a two-
way process, with, in most cases, the parents taking the greater responsibility.
But, in fact, there is a change in the balance of caring as children move into
and through their teens. In the early teens, there is no doubt that usually parents do far more of the caring for their children than the other way round. As
children move through their teens, not always but often, they start to take an
interest in the welfare of their parents. This happens especially when parents
are ill, when they are not getting on together, and when they, the parents, are
facing crises in their own lives.

But sometimes there is more than a change in the caring balance, there is
instead a complete reversal of the expected roles. In the 1990s, interest grew in
the situation of 'young carers'. A survey carried out in the middle of that
decade revealed that there were 50 000 children and young people in the UK,
mainly in their early and mid-teens, mostly looking after a sick parent, though
some were responsible for brothers and sisters, or other relatives. A 16-year-
old young man said in an interview: *'I empty her commode, do the kitchen,
washing up, most of the times I cook dinner … collect her money from the social
security, order her prescriptions, go down doctor's, get a prescription, then go
down chemist—fetch tablets—bring them back, go down shop. Or if she's in the
bath, just wash her hair or something when she can't do it herself. Stuff like that.
Or at night time—because she has trouble getting out of a chair—so I have to lift
her up and put her on the settee to go to sleep, just stuff like that'.*

A 14-year-old girl said 'Instead of our Dad looking after us (following a major stroke) it has changed and now we have to look after him. We have to cook, wash, clean, and do most of the household jobs for both him and ourselves. When we want to go out with friends, our Granny has to look after him'.

What is a 'young carer'? Blackwell's Encyclopaedia of Social Work defines a young carer as 'someone under 18 who carries out, on a regular basis, significant or substantial caring tasks and assumes a level of responsibility that would usually be associated with an adult'. There is an assumption here that we know how to divide tasks up into those adults should do and those that adolescents should be allowed to do. In fact, most young carers want to care for their parents or other family members. They wish to be better supported and, in general, they need much more information, financial help, and emotional support than they get. Exactly whether young carers should have all the responsibility of care removed from them or whether their role should be acknowledged and they should be encouraged to continue with better support is a contentious issue and one to be decided on an individual basis. But what is clear is that when circumstances arise that require those in their early and mid-teens to take responsibility, many of them do remarkably well caring for those who, traditionally, are expected to look after them. There are lessons here for those who find it difficult to acknowledge the competence of young people of this age. After all, young carers are not selected because of their caring competence. They just find themselves having to care.

3.16 Arguments between parents, separation, and divorce: the right of children to be heard

Young carers take responsibility for their parents' care. They have some degree of power in this situation and, broadly speaking, they exercise it well. In other situations, in contrast, they are most inappropriately disempowered. Imagine a group of four adults living in a house, leading a communal existence, eating together, talking over their lives together. Over a few weeks or months, imagine that two of them start to shout and scream at each other, creating an appalling atmosphere. The other two would either quietly leave or, if they couldn't, perhaps because they were tied up financially in the house, they would feel the need to have a say in what was going on. 'Look, you two', they might say, 'we live here too. We need to know what is going on. Can you cool it or sort things out some other way, and if either of you is thinking of leaving, please could you give us some notice, because we have to make arrangements too, you know. We are very fond of you both, but this can't go on'. Children are in exactly this situation when their parents argue and, on occasion, separate and then divorce. Children cannot leave. Their feelings are emotionally more intense than would be the case with the four adults I've imagined. After all, they have known their parents since birth.

In the UK, around one in four children has experienced the divorce or separation of their parents by the age of 16 years and an additional number of children are affected by the breakdown of the relationship of their unmarried parents. Many more, though possibly not as many as used to be the case before divorce became easier, have their lives made miserable by constant arguments between parents.

Traditionally, family life is a private matter and the degree to which parents consult their children is left very much up to them. When one or both parents wish to divorce, until recently it was still left very much up to parents to what degree their children's views were heard. Now it is becoming officially recognized that young people should be consulted in these circumstances and that existing arrangements for doing so are unsatisfactory. It is dangerous to assume that parents will always act responsibly with regard to their children in these situations. Experience suggests that taking their views into account will lead to better decisions more likely to be adhered to in the longer term.

Yet research findings suggest that children in our society are not accustomed to having their views taken into account in their everyday lives at home and at school. We do not live in a culture that supports participation by children. When children whose parents are divorcing are asked about their experience of being interviewed by outsiders such as Children's Guardians (formerly Court Welfare Officers or Probation Officers), about their views, they are uncomplimentary about it. Professionals are too often seen as being more interested in taking the decisions they think are right than in listening and providing support. They are sometimes perceived to be judgemental and intrusive and many children are not confident their views will remain confidential, something that is crucial for them when they may be critical of one parent without wishing to upset their relationship with that parent.

In the words of a 15-year-old, … 'we are people too and shouldn't be treated like low-lifes just because we are younger. I think kids deserve the same sort of respect that we are expected to give to so-called adults'. As seen in Chapter 1, from the age of around 14 years onwards, young people have a degree of understanding of fairness, justice, the rights of individuals, and so on in many respects equivalent to that of adults. There is therefore no reason to exclude them from family discussions on the grounds they are 'too young to understand'. Children under the age of 14 years may not have the same mature level of understanding, but from the age of three or four years upwards, they can certainly grasp and give a view on most aspects of family life.

The lives of children are profoundly affected when their parents separate. The family finances are likely to be more stretched when they have to cover two households rather than one. The family home may have to be sold, and the children live elsewhere with one or other parent. This may mean a change of school and loss of friends. Visits to the so-called non-resident parent may mean weekends are spent completely differently. Perhaps above all, the emotional lives of children may be completely disrupted when the two people of whom they are most fond cannot bear to live together any more. They are at risk of becoming confused, and at least temporarily depressed.

Now it is possible to exaggerate the effects of separation and divorce on children in the family. Their rates of disturbance are increased, but most children in this situation do not suffer from serious long-lasting emotional or behaviour disorders. But their lives will be disrupted, and they will always think differently of their parents in the future.

The adult world often sees children merely as passive victims in this situation. This is far from the case. In one study of children of divorced parents, nearly half the children who were aged between 7 and 15 years, reported that no one had explained to them what the breakdown of their parent's marriage might mean for them in the future. In contrast, most, not surprisingly, wanted to know what was happening. Some children, often even those who had not reached their teen years, reported they had acted as a source of emotional support for one or both of their parents. Only a little over half reported they had been consulted about arrangements where to live and about possible changes of school. Those who had been consulted reported being more satisfied with the way things had been sorted out.

So there is a good evidence to suggest that, when separation is in the air, those in their teens and younger are often not being consulted about arrangements affecting their lives. As in so many other areas of life, young people in their teens need to be consulted about what is happening and, where this is possible, as it often will be, for their views to be taken into account when decisions affecting their lives are made. At one point it seemed as if there would be legislation arising from the 1995 Family Law Act making it obligatory for children to be consulted in these situations, but this law has never been implemented.

3.17 How policy makers can make life easier for parents of teenage children

In this chapter, I have tried to show that happiness and fulfilment in the teen years and beyond is more likely to occur if the young are empowered from an early age. This happens during the development of 'attachment', when notice is taken of how children are feeling. It happens if, as they get older, they are listened to, given an increasingly powerful voice by authoritative parents, and gradually enter into decision-making as equal partners with their parents in democratic families. Growing up inevitably involves frequent experience of differences of opinion between people who love each other. Because this initially occurs entirely in the family, it promotes negotiating skills to be formed that are essential for healthy development.

Some parents and children seem to take to negotiation naturally; others have much greater problems. For those who find negotiation more problematic, the social situation in which they live can contribute to their difficulties or make it easier to overcome them. Policy makers can try to ensure that the circumstances in which the young in their teens and their families live are as favourable for healthy development as possible.

3.18 How can society make it easier for parents and their teenage children to negotiate successfully?

Reducing poverty. In other chapters, I discuss the effect of poverty and income inequality in increasing the likelihood of depression, violence and delinquency, drug taking, overweight and obesity, and educational failure. Here I shall just briefly touch on the effect of poverty on child rearing and family relationships. We all know that money and material possessions bring no guarantee of health or happiness. Further, there are many problems from which young people suffer, including sexual abuse and anorexia, which do not occur particularly among the poor. But authoritarian parenting and the extremes of such parenting, especially the physical abuse of children and those in their teens in the family is very strongly linked to poverty, unemployment, and overcrowded housing conditions.

Though many cope remarkably well, it is extraordinarily difficult for unemployed, depressed parents, living in poverty, lacking hope or any sort of positive expectations for the future, to find the energy or motivation to negotiate with their teenage children. Instead they are inevitably more likely than those living in more affluent circumstances to let their children get on with their lives, unmonitored and unsupervised. When things go wrong as they inevitably sometimes do, parental reactions are likely to be heavy and punitive. Parents are indeed blamed for this. But it is so much easier to negotiate in better-off families when there is more time and, more often, a quiet place to talk. It is so much easier to those in their teens to cool off after an argument with their parents when they have a separate room to go to.

So successful government efforts to reduce poverty, improve employment prospects, and ensure decent housing with sufficient space for the young to enjoy some degree of privacy will promote attunement in infancy, authoritative parenting in childhood and the early teen years, and family democracy in the mid- and late teens—all desirable ingredients for a better future for both parents and their children.

Similarly, government does have some power to reduce the mismatch between the intellectual competence of the young and their financial dependence. This mismatch gives rise to tensions that many families find difficult to sort out amicably in a way that preserves the self-esteem of young people. Giving the unemployed young in their late teens some degree of financial independence by providing them with an entitlement to benefits as well as releasing university students from the payment of fees and entitling them to interest-free loans would go far to reduce family tensions arising from this situation.

Community development involving young people. I shall discuss the need to help young people to feel part of the communities in which they live and to make sure there are sufficient leisure facilities available to them in some detail in Chapter 11. Here it is only necessary to point out that where families feel part of a local community, supported by other people living close by, it will be easier for family members to negotiate successfully among themselves. When a local community is fragmented and disorganized, the young with problems will find others who are disaffected living in their neighbourhoods. Violence against people in their own communities and involvement in heavy drug use may then follow. Government initiatives to support local communities in setting up supportive networks involving both young people and their parents will make it harder for young people to 'take off' when there are family arguments and much easier for democratic parenting to develop. Further, I shall discuss in Chapter 10 that there is a real need to improve the availability and accessibility of leisure facilities, preferably for a mixed age range including those in their early and mid-teens, to help the young get out of the house or flat to somewhere safe when there is unbearable tension between them and their parents.

Reduction of violence in the community. The acceptance of physical violence and verbal humiliation in our society makes it much easier for parents to resort to such methods when they know they are so widely acceptable. This subject is discussed in more detail in Chapter 5. Here it is only necessary to say that the use of physical force by parents does nothing to encourage the sort of negotiation known to be linked to better outcomes for those in their teens. Ways in which society can reduce the widespread acceptability of violence as a means of reaching resolution when conflicts arise are discussed in more detail in the later chapter. They include banning or criminalizing the use of physical punishment by parents so that the young do not model themselves on the notion that physical power decides who wins when conflict arises, treating domestic violence as a crime rather than as a private matter between individuals, reducing media content involving violent methods of conflict resolution, especially in television programmes, videos, and computer games aimed at younger children (so that by the time they reach their teens, the young are at lower risk of using such methods themselves), and banning the sale of toy guns and other toys or games with violent content for the same reason.

Prohibiting television and other commercial advertisement to under 12s. A potent source of tension between parents and their teenage children is linked to the wish of the young to purchase more than the family can afford. The commercial manipulation of those in their teens by creating desires for material possessions such as expensive items of clothing is unavoidable in the predominantly materialist society in which we live. By the time they reach their teens, the young are conditioned to react to commercial advertisements by wishing to purchase with minimal reflection. If their exposure to such advertisement was delayed until their teens, it would be possible for them to have built up a more critical approach to advertisement and thus be in a better position to resist.

Education for parenting. Many parents of young people have been brought up in authoritarian or even abusive families. They often have no other model of bringing up children available to them. They may either replicate the upbringing they have had themselves or react against it so violently that they fail to provide any structure to their children's lives. Finding it impossible to say 'no' may not be quite as pernicious as providing a harsh, physically frightening home to live in, but, as we have seen, it does produce teenage children who have great problems with their friends.

All parents want to do their best for their children, but many just do not have the information they need to help them attune to their infants, provide security and love to their children and reach a stage of democratic family relationships when their children are in their teens. Such information needs to be made available at all times, but pregnancy and the first months of life are probably most crucial in the formation of attitudes. One way to provide such information and the skills to use it helpfully is through parenting workshops, and these are discussed in more detail in Chapter 5. The opportunity for discussion of these issues and the acquisition of negotiating skills in personal relationships can also take place in schools, for example, during Personal, Social, Health Education (PSHE) classes. Sex education in schools containing the opportunity to discuss the intense emotional feelings aroused by sexual activity, as we shall see in Chapter 6, does not, as is sometimes believed, result in earlier sexual activity and may indeed result in delay in the age at which full intercourse occurs. Effective sex education in school may also result in taking some of the heat out of parent–teenage child tensions and make negotiation easier.

Legislating to ensure the voice of the child is heard when parents separate. As we have seen, although parents who are in the process of separation or divorce accept that they need to pay attention to what their children would like, in terms of where they are to live and other crucial aspects of their lives, in practice this often does not happen. Legislation should make it impossible for this situation to continue at least as far as children over the age of 13 are concerned. Where the lives of competent young people/children are so much involved there must be a legal right for them to voice their wishes and for account to be taken of what they say.

Chapter 4

More cheerful than moody

4.1 Introduction

In this chapter I suggest that most of those in their teens are cheerful, happy, and reasonably stable most of the time. As we shall see in more detail later in this chapter, three out of four 13–15-year-olds report that they have never or only occasionally been unhappy over the past years. Contrary to popular belief, young people in their teens, if compared to those in their twenties and thirties, are not moodier or more depressed. Rates of low self-esteem, depression, and suicidal ideas increase in the early teens and then remain stable from about the age of 14 years onwards through the rest of young adulthood and middle age. Thus, as far as mood and mood disorders are concerned, those in their teens are very like those in later adulthood, as they are in so many other aspects of life.

Unfortunately, a number of young people in their teens, like those in later adulthood, *are* severely and pathologically depressed. Milder feelings of depression are very common and part of normal human experience. I go on to suggest that both in the teen years and in later adult life, although genetic influences make some individuals more vulnerable, indeed sometimes much more vulnerable to depression than others, stress plays a major part in triggering depressive episodes. Further, the stresses experienced by those who become depressed either in their teen years or in adult life are often a reflection of a lack of power and control that people have in their family lives or elsewhere. But the reasons for such lack of power and control are not the same in the teen years as they are in later adult life. I then suggest what parents and teachers might do to prevent moodiness and depression in young people in their teens and deal with it when it arises. Finally, I suggest measures those in positions of authority might put in place to increase the control young people in their teens have over their own lives, thus reducing the overall rate of teen depression.

4.2 Moodiness in the teens: a minority experience

It may come as a relief to some and a revelation to others that the teen years are usually a happy time of life for teenagers themselves. The journalists who write about its agonies and its ecstasies have, I suspect, usually had more than their average share of turbulence in their teen years. Further, they are unusually articulate people, whose craft partly involves the creation of dramatic accounts of what might have been rather mundane events. However, as we shall see later in this chapter, the survey evidence does not support the notion that turbulence is a common teenage experience. Further most parents do not find the teen years of their children more stressful than their earlier years. Adolescence has such a bad name that when I talk to parents about their teenage children, and discover that they and their children actually seem to be having a reasonably enjoyable time, they seem almost apologetic. Adolescence has such a bad name it seems that those who pass through it in reasonable tranquillity are thought to have something wrong with them.

The reasons why most teenagers are happy most, though, of course, not all of the time, are not hard to find. Most are loved and made to feel secure by parents who have been looking after them since babyhood. A minority, around one in four, come from homes broken by divorce or separation, but many of those who come from broken homes enjoy a secure home base with their single parent or a step-family in which they feel loved and appreciated.

Though at the beginning of the teens, parents will still be the most important people in their children's lives, by the end of the teens, parents and other important members of the close family will have been partly or sometimes even completely replaced in most of their children's hearts by girlfriends or boyfriends, usually though not always of the opposite sex—young men and women of the same age as themselves who have become the people most significant to them. Parents will still be important but much less so than they were. And most young people have other good friends, who are loyal to them and with whom they have a great deal of fun and enjoyment. They are another source of happiness. Again, contrary to much belief, most teenagers enjoy not only the social side of school, though this is often the main source of pleasure, but at least some of the lessons, usually those they are best at. Then there are the many fun activities often shared with friends; gossip, music, television, videos, computer games, shopping and window shopping, going to cafes and pubs, sport, discos and clubbing, as well as even the occasional outing with one or both of their parents. Combined with all this is the fact that, although many would say they could do with more money, most of this age group do have enough to spend to enjoy themselves at least at weekends. That is, of course, very much not the case for a substantial minority living in families on low incomes in areas of high unemployment where they cannot get work themselves.

So it is not surprising that there is a systematic evidence suggesting most young people in their teens do not experience misery and distress of depth or significance. In a nationwide survey carried out in the UK in 1999, quoted in the last chapter, nearly 2500 parents were asked about their child as to whether a statement that their 13–15-year-old child was 'Often unhappy, down-hearted, or tearful' was Not True, Somewhat True, or Certainly True. Teachers and children themselves were asked the same question. The statement was marked as Not True for about three out of four girls and about four out of five boys by parents, teachers, and those in the early teens themselves. Only about one in thirty parents, teachers, or children themselves said that this statement was Certainly True. More worryingly, about one in five, somewhat more girls than boys, and somewhat more children than their parents and teachers, said the statement was Somewhat True.

Grant is a 14-year-old boy who gets a lot of fun out of life. He is not brilliant at school, but gets by in most subjects and it is thought he will make six GCSEs at Grades C or D. He is a good footballer and is popular for this reason and by virtue of the fact that he is easy going and not easily upset. He has two good friends whom he sees once during the week and at the weekend. His parents split up when he was five years old, and he does not see his father. But his mother remarried after about two years and he gets on well with his stepfather, who is also a football fanatic.

Cheryl is a 13-year-old girl who is more easily upset, especially since her periods started a year ago. Her parents tend to bicker about money and she can't bear it when they do. All the same, she has a group of friends whose company she enjoys. She has a 'best friend', Sandy, a year older than herself, but is worried she is going to become less close to her as she has started to go out with boys. Sandy has reassured her that this will not happen as there are all sorts of things she would never talk about to boys that she wants to talk to Cheryl about. Cheryl is doing well at school where it is thought she will obtain excellent grades when she takes her GCSEs. Cheryl thinks of herself as a happy girl, as do her parents, though the fact that she is easily upset means that her mood is, in fact, quite fragile.

4.3 When teens compare themselves with others

The same story emerges when one looks at whether teenagers think of themselves as really worthwhile, rubbish, or somewhere in between. How do they, in general, regard themselves in comparison with others? A large number of studies have been carried out in recent years on the self-esteem of those in their teen years. A typical questionnaire contains a series of contrasting statements about how children or young people might think about themselves. One example of a pair of statements is 'Some kids are happy with themselves as a person' and 'Other kids are not so happy with themselves'. Another is 'Some kids are popular with others their own age' and 'Other kids are not very popular' and another pair go 'Some kids wish they look different' and 'Other kids like the way they look'. When they complete questionnaires like this, young people are asked whether the positive or negative statements are 'Really True for Me' or 'Sort of True for Me'. In a study of nearly 4000 Scottish children and adolescents, those in their teens generally thought of themselves just slightly more positively than they thought about 'most kids'. Most boys think of themselves as definitely more athletic than 'most kids'. Though to a lesser degree than boys, girls also think of themselves as definitely better than 'most kids' in most areas of life, at school, in their relationships, and in their behaviour, but they think a good deal less well when it comes to their own appearance or athletic ability. Overall boys score higher on self-esteem than do girls. This might be because boys are just more optimistic and well-adjusted or, just as likely, because girls have a more realistic view of themselves. In any event, having reasonably high self-esteem is not a major problem for most young people of this age.

4.4 **Stress and distress do rise once the teens are reached**

The fact that most in their teens lead a reasonably happy existence, does not by any means rule out the possibility that, at the beginning of the teens, there is an increase in the amount of misery and unhappiness experienced at this time of life. Around one in twenty children before puberty experiences great distress for weeks at a time during any one year. This figure increases to around one in three or four in the teens. But it is important to stress that this still means that two out of three or three out of four teenagers are not affected in this way, even though the rate of unhappiness has greatly increased from before to after puberty. Though they may generally be happy, many young people in their teens do not find life easy, and the strain begins to show as soon as they reach puberty. Upsetting events such as rejection, frustration, loss, or disappointment produce sadness, misery, and irritability in people of all ages. Such feelings may last anything from a couple of hours to several days. A number of studies have looked at the way this 'distress experience' changes as children develop and move into adolescence. It turns out that its frequency increases markedly at the beginning of adolescence. When asked how often they feel sad and miserable, younger children, who have not reached their teens, say they have these feelings much less frequently than do adolescents. In one well-known study, only about one in ten 11-year-olds said they felt sad and miserable quite a lot or nearly all the time compared to nearly one in three of the same children once they had reached 14 years.

4.5 Levels of distress remain at the same level in the twenties and beyond

The experience of distress remains at roughly the same level throughout the teens, but it is not a special feature of this time of life. Though they usually show it in a less dramatic fashion, young adults report such feelings at roughly the same frequency as do those in their teen years. People aged 20–25 years experience sadness, misery, and irritability just as much as do those in their teens. To some degree and in some respects, the feelings of distress do very gradually become less frequent after that.

4.6 Clinical depression increases at puberty and remains high in adult life

Clinical depression is an extreme form of distressed mood. As the label suggests, it is a clinical syndrome differing from the distress experience mainly in its seriousness. Like older people, the young who show it are seriously affected and cannot lead a normal life. They are less able to study or carry out their work. They do not want to see their friends. Their family and social lives are significantly impaired. They are much more likely to harm themselves, and when they do, if they survive, they say afterwards that they wanted to end their lives and to take precautions to ensure they are left to die. While the 'distress experience' lasts only a few hours or at the most a few days, young people who have the 'depressive syndrome' remain affected for weeks or months. They blame themselves for what they have done in the past and see no hope for the future. They think other people regard them as useless, unattractive, and unlovable when, in fact, this is not the case.

The best estimates suggest that about one or two in a hundred children show such clinical depression before puberty, but the rate trebles or quadruples to around one in twenty during adolescence. So, compared with younger children, teenagers are not only more likely to suffer the distress experience, but, in addition, they are much more likely to show clinical depression. Unlike the distress experience, which remains stable in frequency once adult life is reached, the frequency of clinical depression actually continues to go up in adulthood. This is especially the case in women. Though before puberty the number of boys and girls show roughly equal amounts of clinical depression, once adolescence is reached, girls become more affected and this gender difference reaches a peak in middle-aged women among whom as many as one in ten is clinically depressed.

The depressive syndrome and the distress experience tend to have different causes. While both are usually triggered by unpleasant events, genes are likely to be more important in influencing the likelihood of clinical depression. Often, though by no means always, there is at least one close relative who has suffered from clinical depression. Though this is less usual, the young person who is clinically depressed is also more likely to have been physically or sexually abused or neglected in earlier life.

4.7 Suicidal attempts reach adult levels in the teen years and then remain high

In England, each year about 7 or 8 in every 1000 girls aged between 15 and 19 years, and about 2–3 in every 1000 boys of this age make suicidal attempts, mainly by taking an overdose of tablets. This means that every day about 45 girls or young women and about 20 boys or young men are seen in Accident and Emergency Departments, somewhere in the country, having taken an overdose. Suicidal attempts begin to occur in girls round about the age of 10 years and reach their peak around 17 years. There is then a very slow decline throughout young adulthood and middle age. In Western Europe, for example, every year nearly 3 in every 1000 young women aged between 15 and 24 years harm themselves, usually by taking an overdose. But well over 2 in every 1000 in older age groups of people aged 25–34. More than one in every thousand 35–44-year-olds take overdoses each year.

What these rather detailed statistics reveal is that although taking an overdose is thought to be very much an adolescent problem, in fact it occurs quite commonly in older people too. Many might think that older people who take overdoses are behaving in an 'adolescent' manner. This way of using the term 'adolescent' is a form of insult, a practice I have deplored in Chapter 1, and it does not alter the fact that overdosing is by no means confined to those in their teens.

4.8 Suicide rises sharply in the early teens and reaches adult levels by the late teens

The same pattern occurs with suicide. It is extremely unusual for a child under the age of 14 years to commit suicide. The official figures suggest that less than one in a million children aged 10–14 years end their own lives each year, compared to 60 times that number aged 15–19 years. By the end of the teens the rate of suicide has more or less stabilized and remains the same throughout the whole of adult life, perhaps with a slight increase in the elderly. So, as far as suicidal behaviour is concerned, 14-year-olds are then, to all intents and purposes, adults. A great deal of publicity was rightly given to the fact that in the 1980s and early 1990s the rate of suicide in boys and young men in their mid and late teens went up to some degree. In the late 1990s, it reached a plateau and then went down slightly. Less publicity was given to the fact that the rate never went as high as that found in young people in later life. In fact in girls and young women of this age it remained substantially lower than that in older people. As far as suicide is concerned, sadly the beginning of the teens also marks the start of this type of adult behaviour, though the frequency remains lower than in older people.

4.9 Why do all forms of distress increase at puberty and remain high throughout life?

Distress and depression are part of normal human experience. Indeed they perform a useful function. The feeling of discomfort they bring may alert us to the need to take action to avoid situations that upset us. The distress that we show when we look unhappy or tearful may help to make other people more sympathetic and comforting to us. So it would be worrying if those in their teens did not show at least some degree of distress and discomfort. But when these emotions become so severe or so long-lasting that they cripple our lives they are doing us no good and are a cause of unnecessary suffering. They may make us a danger to ourselves or to others if we become self-destructive or seriously aggressive. It is clear from the statistics that not only does normal distress and depression increase at puberty and remain high thereafter, but that the same is true of disproportionately severe emotional reactions of every type. Why does this happen?

The obvious reason is that it has something to do with the physical changes that occur at puberty, especially the rise in hormone levels. After all, the most obvious feature distinguishing children from adolescents is their sexual development. In both boys and girls, puberty is a time when there is a massive increase in the amounts of circulating sex hormones, especially oestrogen and testosterone. Investigators have therefore naturally turned their attention to the possible role of hormones causing sadness, misery, and clinical depression. Do hormones make us depressed? In general, as psychologist Christy Miller Buchanan and her colleagues have shown, the results have been firmly negative.

There is some suggestion that a rapid increase in secretion of estrogens in girls are linked to depressive feelings. This is in contrast to adult women where low levels of estrogen are more often found with depression. Mostly though the links between hormone levels and mood are very weak.

There is a popular idea that adolescents are at the mercy of a torrential outpouring of sex hormones that turns them into creatures constantly palpating with uncontrollable desire. Indeed, the most comprehensive scientific review of the subject is titled 'Are adolescents victims of their raging hormones?' But the review concludes that once girls have had their first half a dozen periods and a regular cycle has been established, hormone levels are pretty much the same as those of adult women. Further, apart perhaps from mood changes occurring in teenagers and adults before their periods, there is no evidence that their moods go up or down depending on their hormone levels. The same is broadly true of boys. So the explanation for the rise in sadness, misery, and clinical depression in early adolescence is unlikely to lie with hormones.

Although the rise in emotional distress is therefore unlikely to be due to a direct effect of the increase in hormone levels, this does not rule out the possibility that sexual feelings are involved in the change that occurs. After all, loss is more poignant and agonizing when it involves someone to whom one is sexually attached. But even this does not seem a totally convincing explanation. Girls in their teens form deep attachments to their friends that are usually non-sexual in nature. They are desperately upset if, for some reason or other, for example because a close friend rejects them or leaves the district, the relationship is broken.

4.10 **Competent but powerless: the shared predicament of teens and adults**

When vulnerable individuals suffer disappointment, the risk of inappropriately severe distress or clinical depression is reduced if they can actively and energetically do something about whatever it is that is causing them grief. If they have control over their own lives they are much more likely to be able to do this. The experiments with rats carried out in the 1960s by Morton Seligman, showed how rats went into states of withdrawal if, no matter how they behaved, they were frustrated in obtaining food in ways that had previously met with success. These experiments have relevance to this day. Seligman called the situation that produced this state of withdrawal in rats 'learned helplessness'. It remains highly relevant to our understanding of emotional upset once the teen years have been reached, not only in the teens, but throughout the whole of adult life.

As seen in Chapter 1, by the early teens, the young have, in many respects, reached adult levels of intelligence. Their capacity for reasoning is as good as it will ever be. They think as clearly as adults. In some respects, especially in the use of new technology to gain access to information, they are streets ahead of most people older than themselves. It has been said that everyone over the age of twenty is an immigrant in the new world of information technology. Only the teens have been born into this world; the rest of us have to struggle to feel part of it. So it is natural that those who have reached their teens should feel distressed and frustrated when their competence is not recognized. When young people reach this age, for the first time they experience simultaneously a sense of power and an incapacity to use their new found competence. The frustration and the potential for the creation of distress this brings will remain with them for the rest of their lives. We all have to live with it.

What the young do lack, it will be pointed out, is the experience to deal with the new situations with which life presents them. They may be very clever, but they don't know how to use their cleverness because they haven't lived long enough to learn from their mistakes. There is, of course, a great deal of truth in this. But distress is related much more to the way those in their teens think about themselves than the way adults think of them. Many in their teens recognize, in some circumstances, the need to gain experience before they can shoulder the responsibility of taking decisions for themselves. But frustration and distress, sometimes deep distress, arise when the young feel, often quite reasonably, that they are better judges of their own competence and previous experience than those who deny them the right to be heard, let alone act on their own behalf.

4.11 The special features of powerlessness in the teens

Every phase of life has its own special reasons for the experience of powerlessness. The young mother in her late twenties or early thirties, sitting at home with a crying, unhappy baby, may feel not only unable to quieten her child but also separated from her friends who might support her. The middle-aged man, threatened with redundancy in a failing firm in which he is only a middle manager, may feel he can do nothing to protect his job. A civil servant aged 60 years, who has just reached retirement age after a lifetime of dedicated public service in which she has not had time to develop other interests, may feel seriously distressed by her special life situation. A man of eighty, who has always been active and healthy, may feel utterly helpless, cut off, and depressed by virtue of failing vision and increasing deafness. Each of these is at risk of depression because of a social situation characteristic of the phase of life they have reached. Similarly, those in their teens are vulnerable to distress and depression because of their special life situation. In fact, many in their early and even mid and late twenties now share the same social situation as those in their teens. What are the features of life in the teens and often for those in their twenties that are specially stressful?

In other chapters, I discuss the different ways in which the young can feel either empowered or disempowered in family life, in school, and in the neighbourhood or community. Here, mainly by providing some examples, I point to the ways in which disempowerment in these different structures or circumstances leads to distress and depression.

Let us begin with the family.

Jennifer is a 14-year-old girl who lives with her mother on an inner city estate in the north of England. She has a close friend at school with whom she wants to go on a school trip to France at the end of the winter term, in six months time, with the rest of her class. Her mother says she cannot afford to pay for her, but Jennifer has worked out that if she takes a job delivering newspapers for three months in the holidays she will be able to pay for herself. Her mother says she is not happy for her to take this job because she does not want her to be out first thing in the morning. She is worried she will be molested. Jennifer is physically a large girl, and thinks she can look after herself. She knows the area is not a dangerous one. However her mother's word has to carry as the newsagent will not employ anybody of Jennifer's age without parental permission. Three years ago, Jennifer would have found it easier to accept her mother's decision, but now she has cottoned onto the fact that the real reason her mother does not want her to take the job is because she does not like being left alone in the house first thing in the morning. Her mother also has difficulty leaving the flat, even to do the shopping, so Jennifer has to do most of it herself. She cannot talk to her mother about this as her mother would be ashamed and humiliated to have to admit to her problem. Jennifer knows that fear of being alone and of travelling are common problems. She has a friend whose mother has a similar difficulty and who has had some treatment for it. So Jennifer, who has longed for this school journey and planned for it sensibly becomes frustrated and distressed. She feels trapped and cannot think of a way out. She loses concentration at school, and starts not to want to go out herself. She is weepy and unhappy. Eventually her mother suggests that she goes to see the doctor and she does. He gives her tablets, the same ones her mother has received. Her distress deepens.

Jennifer is a competent young person. She understands her mother better than does her mother herself. Yet her age and the fact that she is seen by society as unable to make decisions for herself means that she experiences frustration and a sense of impotence leading directly to distress and depression. Such situations arise not just because of the fact that some parents find it difficult to take the perspective of their children, but because the family as an institution is not set up to allow the young in their teens the autonomy to which their competence should entitle them. This is as much a problem for society as it is for parents. After all, governments and the media constantly berate parents when their children behave badly. The notion that parents should control their teen children better is widespread in our society. It is not surprising that many parents find it hard to give their children responsibility for their actions at a level they can handle.

Fourteen-year-old Carol went to her bedroom at 10 o'clock one evening and took 20 paracetamol tablets. The following morning she did not appear for breakfast and her mother could not rouse her when she went to wake her. The ambulance was called and Carol was taken to the nearest Accident and Emergency Department. She was resuscitated and treated rapidly, so that, as sometimes happens after paracetamol overdosing, liver failure was avoided, and the need for a liver transplant did not arise. (It is not widely known that paracetamol poisoning following suicidal attempts is the commonest reason for liver transplantation in the UK and by far the commonest reason in teenagers needing such transplants.) She was admitted to an adult ward, where over the next couple of days, a child and adolescent psychiatrist saw her and her parents, both separately and as a family group.

The following story emerged. Carol was an above average student at a mixed comprehensive school with a mainly middle class catchment area. She had fallen in love with an older boy, 17-year-old Joe, who attended the same school, and they had been going around together for about six months. On the evening in question, Joe had been invited to the birthday party of a boy in his form. He had expected to take Carol along, but the party was expected to last until the early hours of the next morning, and Carol's father had always insisted that she be back by midnight. Joe said he would go to the party by himself unless she could stay at least until two in the morning. Carol knew there would be other attractive girls at the party, and Joe would be a catch. She pleaded with her father to be allowed to stay out later but he was adamant. He would not give any reasons. He said it was obvious why a 15-year-old girl should not stay out so late.

The psychiatrist found Carol to be angry, but not clinically depressed. She thought it was a waste of time to talk, though she did say she thought she had been silly to take the tablets and said she would not do it again. Carol's parents were extremely upset, but puzzled how they could have handled the matter differently. Her father, who worked in a bank, after some hesitation, explained that when he was eighteen, his younger sister had become pregnant at the age of sixteen. The father of the child did not want to take any responsibility. His sister had had a termination. The whole matter had caused enormous upset in his family. He made the psychiatrist promise that she would not raise this matter in the family meeting. His sister, Carol's aunt, was now happily married with two children, and would be mortified if Carol knew about her pre-marital pregnancy. Carol's mother, a school secretary, admitted she had difficulty talking to Carol about her periods, let alone sexual matters, and would not be able to talk to her about contraception. She wants to support her husband, but feels for Carol in her predicament. So Carol is caught in a Catch 22 situation, and one that is quite likely to arise again. Should she risk losing her boyfriend, or disobey her parents?

Here we can see how the assumption in family life that young people in their teens should be denied information that is relevant to the way their parents behave leads to their experiencing a sense of impotence followed by distress and depression. Poor communication within families can lead to even more tragic consequences.

Sam was a 14-year-old boy with an attractive, lively, but rather provocative personality, and keen on sport, especially football. He had gone through puberty earlier than nearly all the other boys in his class at school, so that when they transferred to secondary school, he was one of the tallest. But then the others had more than caught up, they had overtaken him, and by fifteen he was almost the smallest boy in the class. This was upsetting for him because he was dropped from the year football team. It had not helped that he had got across the PE teacher because he argued with his decisions and not always in the most tactful way. The PE teacher called him 'titch' or 'titchface' and said that a 5 foot 5 inch centre forward was not what he wanted. Sam lost out socially, and became a bit of a loner. Then he began to become withdrawn and lost interest in school and in his collection of CDs, which had always been his pride and joy. He said he did not want to see his friends, even on those unusual occasions when they did call for him. He went off his food, lost a little weight and his mother took him to the doctor. The doctor examined him and found 'nothing wrong'. The doctor told his mother he was 'going through a phase and this was natural at his age'. He would get out of it. A week later he was found dead, having hanged himself in his bedroom in what was obviously a premeditated act. He had bought a strong rope two days previously.

But this is not the whole story. Alarm bells should have rung. Before Sam was born his father, also a relatively short man who worked as a bus driver, had on two occasions been admitted to hospital. He had been so severely depressed that he was given electroconvulsive therapy. Sam's mother knew about this but it was never talked about in the family, so she had not told the doctor who, in turn, had not asked whether anyone in the family had suffered depression. The doctor had also not seen Sam by himself, when he could have asked more easily about possible suicidal thoughts. The tragedy was avoidable.

This story illustrates some of the main causes of suicide in those in their teens and the way in which the disempowerment of teenagers may be relevant to the tragic outcome. When they are victimized, those in their teens can do much less about it and are more impotent than are adults in a similar situation. In theory, Sam could have told his parents about the way the PE teacher was treating him, but, in fact, he would not have dreamed of doing any such thing. He did not feel empowered to do so. He did not confide any of his troubles to them, and even if he had, they did not have the sense that they could make any difference to the way the school functioned, so they would not have gone up to the school to complain. The second important factor in the suicide is the failure to recognize Sam's depression once it had occurred. He showed all the warning signs of a dangerous level of depression. In an adult, this would have triggered off major concern in the doctor. Yet adolescents are not supposed to get depressed; their signs of distress are invisible. The way adults ignore the signs of depression in the young is another reason for their disempowerment.

We see with Sam a combination of disempowerment at home and at school. Sometimes the problem lies solely in school.

Fourteen-year-old Dave is reasonably bright and doing well at school, but he is very clumsy and overweight and wears glasses. Not surprisingly, he is no good at games. In his inner city comprehensive, bullying is rife, though the teaching staff is in the dark about it and would be horrified if they knew what was going on. Every day on his way home from school Dave is mocked, called names, and pushed around by a group of boys who are in a remedial stream. He spends the afternoon dreading his journey home. His mother, who was deserted by Dave's father when Dave was a baby, is depressed, and Dave does not want to add to her worries by telling her about the bullying. What can Dave do? He can complain to a teacher and risk further intimidation. He can bring himself to tell his mother and add to her worries. He can start a fight and risk being seriously beaten up. He can pretend to have a serious headache or stomach ache and take a few days off school. None of these solutions seems very appealing. Should he take an overdose? If he does, it is quite likely that the predicament in which Dave finds himself will be tackled helpfully from his point of view. The bullying in school will come to light and the authorities may do something about it. Dave's mother may become more sympathetic and able to communicate with him in the future about his worries. In fact, not surprisingly, he becomes quite seriously depressed.

Note again how different is Dave's plight from that of a 25-year-old man who is suffering constant, belittling criticism from his boss at the estate agent where he works. Leaving school is not a possibility for Dave. He attends the only school in the neighbourhood, and anyway he does not really want to leave a school where he is making good progress and the teachers like him. For the man who is unhappy at work, at least if he is relatively young, leaving and finding another job is a real option. One characteristic predicament of those in their teens who make suicidal attempts is that they are trapped in situations from which there is no legitimate escape.

Another problem is the difficulty adolescents have in finding someone to whom they can communicate their worries. As we saw, Dave couldn't talk to his mother and he felt there was no one in school in whom he could confide. He had good mates, but, typically for a boy, there was no one to whom he could tell his story. His lines of support, so important for adults who are at risk for becoming depressed, were non-existent. This was not just Dave's problem. He shares it with most of those in their teens who are bullied in or out of school, or have other depressing experiences to contend with. Parents, even parents with good relationships with their teenage children, just do not seem to know about their depressive feelings. In one study of a group of 16–19-year-old girls and their mothers in which I was involved, hardly any of the mothers knew about the suicidal feelings many of their daughters experienced, and it was not at all uncommon for mothers not even to be aware of the fact that their daughters had actually made suicidal attempts in the past.

In Chapter 9, we shall see how empowering young people in school is the most effective means of preventing bullying. If this approach to bullying is taken, it makes communication between young people and between them and their parents much easier so that if it does occur, there are better means of recruiting help.

4.12 **Boosting confidence in teen children: what parents and teachers can do**

Striking the right balance between being over- and under-confident is a challenge for everybody, not just for those in their teens. We all try to achieve the best balance we can. Under-confidence will mean we cannot use the skills and talents we have; over-confidence will result in upsetting other people and letting them down. Both increase our risk of developing long-lasting distress and depression. For those in their teens, reaching roughly the right balance (and the balance is never perfect, or, if it is, it won't be for long!) will mean they can feel good, but perhaps not too good about themselves. Such a balance gives them the best chance of using the talents they have to good advantage, having a sense of personal fulfilment, getting on with others, and establishing sound personal characteristics that will serve them well in the future.

For young people in their teens, one of the tasks they face throughout their teen years is to continue to like themselves, to understand themselves, to improve their understanding of others, to develop their talents, to remain energetic, and to think positively about the present and the future. It is worth pointing out that this is a legitimate aim for everybody, including parents of those in their teens, and teachers, whose job is to help them learn. We all, teenagers and adults alike, have to try to like and understand ourselves. Being able to do this while bringing up or teaching teenage children is sometimes not at all easy.

A few principles may be helpful. They need to be combined with those in Chapter 5, where ways of avoiding conflict and dealing with conflict when it arises are discussed. Clearly, success or failure in dealing with conflict will have an effect on a teenage child's self-confidence.

Respecting individuality. As I indicated in the last chapter, it always worries me when parents tell me that they treat all their children the same. Frankly, although I only occasionally admit it, I don't believe them. Children don't allow you to treat them the same. Some are more demanding than others, while some need more coaxing to bring them on. Some need more time; others are more self-reliant. Some need constant encouragement to keep focused; others seem to keep their eye on the ball without any help from anybody. There is plenty of evidence that children are born with different temperaments. Different experiences make them even more different. Anyone with more than one child of their own, knows how their children have been born different and how such differences increase as time goes on.

Finding a lifestyle that gives enough time for your teenager. A small minority of young people seem to be extraordinarily self-reliant even in their early teens. Most need time with their parents to talk about what is happening to them and to get help and advice when faced with the challenges described earlier in this chapter. Parents will find it difficult to do this unless they plan their lives to make sure such time is available. Busy jobs, the demands to meet financial commitments, relationship problems of their own, may all make finding time difficult. But parents who, before they take on new commitments, think about what this extra task is going to do to their family life seem to make better decisions. This will be much harder for those who are in difficult financial circumstances or are living without friends of family to support them. This is why the relief of poverty and the provision of support to lone parents are important components of policies to promote positive development of children of all ages.

Providing a model of love, caring, and good communication. If only we could! But we do need to recognize at least to ourselves that children learn less from what their parents and teachers tell them to do, more from how they actually see them behave. If children see their parents showing affection to each other, communicating well, and sorting out their differences, even important differences about which they feel passionately, in an amicable manner, they will learn important lessons how to manage their own lives.

Noticing what other parents do. Parents who have friends they can talk to and confide in with children the same age as theirs, or preferably just a little bit older, will learn from the successes and mistakes of others. It is, of course, often easier to see how other people should be managing their lives than managing one's own.

Trying to understand the world from the viewpoint of your teenager. Young people of teen age often say that parents do not understand that the world has changed since they, their parents, were teenagers themselves. This is true, but possibly more important is the amount the memories parents have of their own adolescence are distorted by time and wish fulfilment. So one can really only learn about the viewpoint of one's children from listening to them, getting inside their heads, working out what it feels like to be them, making sure one communicates to them with sympathy the understanding one has gained, and checking out with them if one has got it right. If parents do this they are much more likely to find their children do the same for them.

Remembering to tell teenage children you feel pleased with them. Somehow for most of us the impulse to feedback to our children how we feel about them is greater when we are fed up and frustrated than when we are pleased with them. This is clearly the wrong way round, and we need to be constantly aware of the need to give praise where it is due and sometimes when it is only just due. The principle that carrots work better than sticks is so well based on evidence, it is amazing we find it so difficult to put it into practice. Helping the young to feel pleased with themselves is a skill too rarely practiced. It is much more common to hear parents say 'You have only yourself to blame', than 'You have only yourself to feel pleased with'.

Empowering teenage children to the greatest degree possible. If young people are involved in family decision-making and, as discussed in Chapter 9, in decision-making in schools, they are much more likely to live with the consequences even if these are not to their liking. A holiday may go wrong or a purchase may turn out to be ill-advised. In either event, if children have taken part in making the decision, they will react more positively to the experience and be more inclined to make the best of it. They are also more likely to be helpful around the house if they feel that, at least to some degree, the house belongs to them too.

Being sympathetic to reasonably safe experimentation but making it clear that dangerous behaviour is foolish and unacceptable. Many of us spend our whole lives trying out new experiences. Those in teen age perforce have to do this more than most. Teenagers need encouragement to keep their life and relationship experiments reasonably safe, so that their lives or futures are not put in unnecessary danger. But they need parents and teachers who are sympathetic when experiments go wrong. All adults need friends and family who are prepared to do the same for them. In addition, though we may not take their advice, we need people to tell us when they think we are endangering ourselves.

Trying to get help when teenage confidence is lost and it is difficult to know what to do. Some young people in their teens become seriously distressed and depressed even though they have marvellous parents and teachers. An essential ingredient of being a marvellous parent is to be able to admit when it is necessary to get outside help. It is this situation that is addressed in the next section.

4.13 Helping distress and depression: the role of parents and teachers

Distress and depression are part of the human condition. Those in their teens are human beings too, so parents and teachers must expect them to show these feelings like everyone else. When children are young, parents feel responsible for their children's moods. The mother of a miserable three-year-old feels bound to find out why her child is unhappy and tries to do something about it. She feels somehow responsible. As children move into their teens these feelings of parental responsibility remain, even though they become less appropriate and perhaps, towards the end of the teens, quite inappropriate. Children and young people increasingly have to take responsibility for their own moods and feelings of distress. All the same, for most parents, because they have developed a habit of caring, there is often no point at which they can stop themselves wishing to relieve distress in their children. Many teachers feel the same about children in their classroom.

Ordinary sadness and distress in the teen years usually last no more than a few hours. Even when the young have suffered what they feel to be a serious loss, they usually last no more than a few days. When young people in their teen years are persistently unhappy over weeks, it is time to take note. If they are withdrawn and miserable, it is easy to recognize something is wrong. But disruptive and difficult behaviour may also be a sign of distress and this is harder to recognize. Further, disruptive children have more than their fair share of depression because they are frequently criticized and, as they see it, humiliated.

Another sign of depression in young people is a lack of pleasure and interest in ordinary, everyday activities. They may say they feel bored. Such 'boredom' is not usually a sign of depression, but it is quite likely to be so when young people have the opportunity to do things they normally enjoy, but seem not to want to participate. If they don't want to see their friends or they lack interest in their favourite hobbies or sports, these can be warning signs, as can difficulty in getting off to sleep or waking in the night. Many teenagers have difficulty getting up in the morning. If they have been up late or parents know the day holds challenges for them they would prefer not to face, this is very understandable and cannot be put down to depression. But they may have been to bed at a reasonable time and still be irritable and unhappy in the morning. That is more worrying.

Of course, the most worrying sign that serious depression is present is when suicidal ideas are expressed. These can range from feelings that life is not worth living or that it would be better to be dead, through to definite expression of suicidal intentions or even to a suicidal attempt. The tone of voice in which these ideas are spoken about is significant. Younger children may express such ideas rather casually because they know they can send adults into a panic this way. But, in general, suicidal ideas in those of teen age must be taken very seriously.

By far the most helpful way parents and teachers can help distressed and depressed young people is by finding time to listen, and *really* listen to them. This is not as easy as it sounds. If their children are depressed, it is not at all unlikely that parents themselves may be wrapped up in their own problems (perhaps the death of a relative or friend or a marriage problem). They may feel helpless and useless in the face of someone else's despair, just be too busy, or find depression in their child too upsetting to think about. It is much easier for parents to listen once they have recognized why they don't really want to!

Listening to a young person who may be depressed needs dedicated time. So it is important to take the telephone off the hook, switch off the mobile, and find a place where you won't be interrupted. Most young people find it takes time before they can say how they are feeling and what it is that is worrying them. They may never be able to tell an adult, but that doesn't mean adults can't be helpful. By being available and supportive, by not blaming and by avoiding the temptation to cheer up the young person with expressions like 'why don't you just look on the bright side of things' or 'it's really not the end of the world', adults can be really helpful.

Just occasionally, parents and teachers may be able to offer practical help to find a solution to a situation about which the young person is depressed or anxious. Bullying may require a visit to the school by a parent to find out what is going on. Some advice about how to handle a relationship that has gone wrong may be acceptable. Both parents and teachers must be prepared to have their advice ignored without regarding the rejection as a personal affront. It is important to be realistic. Not everything can be changed. It is also important to remember that not all feelings of depression are caused by bad experiences. When other family members have shown depressive tendencies, or there are cycles or swings of mood from depression to elation, or from one bout of severe depression to another, or when depressive moods seem to come and go almost regardless of the occurrence of bad experiences, it is time to think of the influence of genes as one of the causes of depression.

When is professional help needed? Certainly when the depression has not lifted after two to three weeks, when everyday life is being interfered with, when there is severe disturbance of sleep and eating patterns, or (definitely and rapidly) when there are suicidal thoughts or feelings. In all these circumstances the young person should be encouraged to attend a drop-in clinic or centre, or visit the family doctor. If the depression does not lift, then referral to a child and family psychiatric clinic in the case of a young teenager or to a psychiatric clinic for adolescents or young adults for those in their late teens will be the best course of action.

4.14 Boosting self-esteem and reducing depression: what society could do

Reducing poverty and other forms of social disadvantage. Not surprisingly, young people living in families struggling to make ends meet find it hard to achieve an enjoyable quality of life. Much pleasure in life comes from variety of experience, whether this be variety of diet or variety of leisure pursuits. Young people whose families can only afford the same cheap and usually unhealthy meals every day, who cannot afford the bus fare into town to see friends or go window-shopping, who have no privacy in their homes, whose parents cannot find more than a token sum for pocket money, and who cannot find part-time jobs to earn some extra money themselves are condemned to spending time out of school and in school holidays watching television or videos or engaged in other passive activities.

It is not just that poverty makes it much more difficult to achieve an enjoyable quality of life. There is solid evidence that young people living in families who are socially disadvantaged more often report themselves to be miserable and unhappy than those living in comfortably-off families. Interestingly, when it comes to serious depressive disorders, in which genes and chemistry are more important, there is very little, if any, difference between the social groups.

So measures that reduce poverty, improve the housing of those living in the poorest accommodation, enable those in their teens to earn some extra spending money themselves, and improve access to sports clubs and other leisure facilities will improve the enjoyment and self-esteem of the worst off young people and reduce the numbers feeling unhappy, sad, and depressed.

Encouraging harmony in family relationships. Traditionally, family life is a private matter. The idea that the state has any part to play in determining how well family members get on with each other is likely to seem objectionable to many people. Yet the economic costs and suffering to others in society created by the casualties of family disharmony mean that it is not at all unreasonable to consider what society can do to reduce it. Much crime, running away from home and prostitution, as well as the depressive feelings that are very much part of these types of behaviour, arise out of domestic violence or less extreme forms of family disharmony.

There is in fact a fair amount that government and local authorities can do, and in some cases are already doing, though often rather ineffectually, to reduce family disharmony. *Supporting parenting programmes* such as the sort of parenting programmes discussed in Chapter 5 that teach better ways of dealing with conflict than verbal abuse and physical assault are increasingly being taken up and should be universally available. If parents can communicate their feelings to each other and to their children and, in addition, they can be helped to listen to their children, especially when their children are unhappy or angry, this will reduce family quarrels and arguments and increase the self-esteem of the children and reduce their risk of depression. *The promotion of sensible drinking patterns,* as considered in Chapter 7, would have a similar effect, for much quarrelling and domestic violence takes place when one or both parents is drunk.

Making child development and the stimulation of emotional intelligence a compulsory part of the school curriculum is discussed in Chapter 9. It is relevant here because of the positive effect this would have on the self-esteem of children and young people. There are other aspects of the school curriculum and of school life over which the government and local authorities have influence that also have a significant effect on the self-esteem and rates of depression of young people. The current emphasis on the achievement of decent standards of literacy and numeracy is, of course, highly desirable so that children can grow up employable and be able to play a full part in life after school. But there needs to be more to school life than reaching national standards. Encouragement to read books for enjoyment, to write creatively, to take part in drama, and to listen to and make music are all calculated to improve the quality of the lives of young people and reduce their risk of depressive feelings. These are activities that bring out the individuality of young people. Making space for them in the school curriculum provides essential ingredients in the promotion of self-esteem.

Helping parents and teachers identify depression and suicidal ideas. Despite the best efforts of parents and teachers, some young people will inevitably become depressed, some seriously so. Government and local authorities can try to ensure that everyone in the population, but especially parents and teachers, are able to recognize the signs of depressive disorder and take appropriate action. Noticing depression, not just in young people who are sad and withdrawn, but also those who are angry and aggressive, is the first step in taking effective action. Ensuring that parents and those professionally involved with young people can recognize depression and suicidal ideas and know what to do once they have done so, is a duty still largely neglected by those in authority.

Making sure mental health services are available to those young people who need them. There are now effective ways of helping most young people who suffer from depressive disorders and suicidal ideas. They need to be readily available, without long waiting lists and be able to react sensitively to the needs of young people. There is good evidence that in the UK at least there are many parts of the country where such services are seriously inadequate in both these respects.

Chapter 5

Everyday hassles, conflict, and crime

5.1 Introduction

In this chapter I shall discuss first, just how true is the commonly held belief that when children reach their teens they become more disobedient and difficult in the family. I shall then look at the likelihood of they becoming involved in criminal activity in the neighbourhood. The evidence shows, as we shall see later in this chapter, that most teenaged young people do not show aggressive behaviour in their families nor do most become involved in crime. The majority are generally obedient at home, though they may well become involved in minor hassles with other family members, especially their parents. They are also largely law-abiding outside the home. The MORI 2002 Youth Survey found that three in four young people aged 11–18 years said they had not committed an offence in the last 12 months. However, a sizeable minority do start to show antisocial behaviour for the first time once they reach their teens. In addition, a much smaller minority, who have been seriously problematic since early childhood, continue to cause great trouble in their teens. A different approach is required to prevent and deal with each of these two groups. For the first, attention needs to be focused on the ways in which they are treated as young children when their problems first develop. Once they reach the teen years their problems are difficult and expensive, though not impossible to resolve. I shall suggest that the size of the larger problematic group, whose antisocial behaviour is limited to the teen years and early twenties could be reduced if the competence of those in this age group was better acknowledged and they were more strongly empowered.

5.2 The myth of the increasingly disobedient teenager

As seen in Chapter 3, when their children approach the teens, the questions parents ask themselves about the future often revolve around control and discipline. This is understandable. Newspaper and magazine articles and a flood of television programmes, soaps as well as documentaries, suggest that the teen years are a time of inevitable and serious conflict between parents and their children. So parents wonder whether, when their children reach teen age, they will start staying out all night, go in for bizarre hairstyles or clothes, cut school and give up their studies, start mixing with friends who are delinquent and using drugs, eventually be in trouble with the police themselves.

Young people in their teens often behave in ways their parents would prefer they didn't. Mostly this involves what their parents, though certainly not the young themselves, regard as unconventional aspects of lifestyle involving, for example, clothes, hair style or colour, metallic adornments or preferred music. But there is a very important difference between unconventionality and anti-social behaviour. Wearing outrageous clothes is a different matter from stealing them from a shop. Dancing to an aggressive beat is very different behaviour from beating up old ladies. There is one important exception, the use of illicit drugs, when this distinction is a good deal less clear. Here conventional behaviour may indeed be illegal and therefore technically antisocial. I shall discuss this further in Chapter 7.

But the majority of those in their teens, around three in every four, do not show anything that could really be regarded as significantly antisocial behaviour. This is in marked contrast to the image that the adult population has of this age group. Many adults admit that when they see a group of young male teenagers approaching them, their first thought is that they are about to be attacked. So powerful is the influence of the stereotype of the violent teenager in our minds that the fact we are not attacked does not seem to make us any less frightened the next time the experience occurs.

This does not mean that life with young people in their teens is always smooth. The occurrence of hassles between family members ensures this is not the case. But, as we shall see, these minor disagreements are not just irritating occurrences, they are learning experiences for both the young and their parents.

5.3 **Everyday hassles**

Children and adolescents are no different from adults in that they learn by testing their beliefs and actions against those of other people. The difference is that in the family they have a built-in system to make sure this happens. Everyday hassles or minor conflicts are an essential part of this learning process. Such hassles begin in infancy and they really never end so long as family members live together.

Growing up and learning through minor conflict is therefore a lifelong process. The teen years are important in this process, but so are other phases of life. Whenever it occurs, conflict is sorted out or sometimes not sorted out by negotiation. A 2-year-old boy decides he does not like green vegetables in whatever form they are served up to him. Spinach, spring greens, broccoli, peas are all unacceptable. His mother insists. His mouth closes firmly or, if a morsel finds its way through his pursed lips, he rapidly spits it out. His mother may attempt negotiation. She may offer pudding only on condition he finishes his greens. She may or may not be successful. Either way he has learned a lesson in the gaining of independence and in his sense of personal autonomy. His mother may have learned something about the release of power.

As psychologist Laurence Steinberg has shown, everyday hassles revolve around a variety of issues where the teenage young are involved. The increased interest in personal appearance means that there is more often a queue for the use of the bathroom. Parents may have views on the undesirability of certain friends and may try to exert unwanted influence. Clothes and hairstyle may meet with disapproval. The time teenagers are expected to return home in the evening may require negotiation and there may be arguments when the agreement is broken. Bedrooms may be left in a mess. Music may be played at what parents regard as objectionable volume. The discovery by a parent of a packet of condoms accidentally left in the pocket of a jacket put aside for cleaning may lead to a heated discussion. Homework not completed, television incessantly watched, obsession with computer games, and difficulty getting up in the morning are other frequent areas of disagreement.

Such hassles between parents and their children have always begun before the teen years, and they rarely stop when the teen years end. A 24-year-old postgraduate student may take out a bank loan against his parents' wishes when they have refused him money themselves, or he may negotiate with them and reach some form of compromise. A 22-year-old daughter, still living at home, may introduce a new young man to her parents at breakfast and find herself attacked for not warning them this was going to happen. In each of these circumstances, a process of negotiation is likely to ensue, very similar to that occurring when their child was in the teens.

At all ages the sorting out of disagreements results in at least a temporary change in relationships. From the child or young person's point of view there may be a step towards the making of independent decisions or a temporary halt in the process. Either way, the sorting out of the daily hassles that form part of everyday family life provides a positive learning experience for both parents and their children. There is evidence that, as children move from early to mid-adolescence, arguments become less frequent as children become more competent in decision-making and parents develop a more realistic appreciation of their children's limitations and capacities. It has been suggested that such hassles are necessary if the young are to achieve independence.

There may be some truth in that, though many young people seem to achieve independence without having ill-tempered arguments with their parents.

There is a sizeable minority where such generally happy family relationships do not exist. Here there may be violent conflict, long periods of not speaking, unwillingness to accept authority, or deep resentment that authority has been ignored. Because psychiatrists and psychologists see families with these types of problem and do not see those where amicable resolution occurs, they sometimes reach the conclusion that violent conflict is the rule in family life with the teens rather than the exception. On the contrary, survey evidence of families in the general population makes it quite clear this is not the case. Following relatively minor disturbances or perturbations in the family when disagreements occur, friendly relationships are usually restored fairly quickly. Later in this chapter, I shall discuss the ways much more serious disharmony arises and how it is handled.

5.4 **Peer pressure and conflicts**

One of the most common sources of conflict or daily hassles between parents and their teenaged children occurs around friendships. From the time they enter infant school, children are influenced in all manner of ways by their peers. Indeed, psychologists such as Judith Rich Harris argue that from this age onwards, children are more influenced by their friends than by their parents, and when it comes to hairstyle, clothes, taste in music, and other aspects of lifestyle, this is certainly the case. But with more fundamental issues, such as moral judgements, the importance given to education, religious beliefs, attitudes to alcohol and drugs, and the level of commitment to other family members, children are more likely to adopt the values of their parents than those of their friends. Indeed, as Dr Ungar, an American psychologist suggests, the evidence suggests that those in their teens choose friends whose values in these respects are similar to their own. When their friends exert pressure on them to behave in particular ways, they are often, though of course by no means always, pushing them in the same directions as their parents.

5.5 **Risk-taking or just learning?**

Before going on to discuss the minority of those in their teens who do become involved in various forms of antisocial activity, what of the commonly held view that those in their teens are 'naturally' risk-takers, reckless, often positively courting danger? How much truth is there in this idea?

In the haste to find bad news about the teens it is often forgotten that adolescence is the healthiest time of life. The death rate is lower than at any other time.

Susceptibility to infection, the bane of the infant and young child has decreased by adolescence because of an increase in immunity, and the risk of developing heart disease or cancer, the great killers of the middle-aged and elderly, is still very low. So the most common causes of serious disability and death that occur in teenagers are accidents and injuries. This is at least partly because other causes of illness and death are so low rather than the rate of accidents is so high. The explanation most frequently put forward for those injuries that do occur is the tendency of the adolescent to take risks. They have a bad reputation for risking their own and other people's lives. But in fact, this is just another way in which adolescents are denigrated and stigmatised.

Activities most commonly regarded as 'risk-taking' are driving dangerously, having unprotected sex or sex with multiple partners, drinking alcohol to excess, cigarette smoking, using illegal drugs, involvement in dangerous sporting activities such as rock-climbing, and, in the United States and other countries, where firearms are so readily available, playing with guns. There is indeed evidence to support the idea that, in many of these activities, the young in their teens do take more risks than people of other ages. But one needs to look at each of them separately to consider whether the teenage years are indeed the most hazardous and, if they are, why this should be. Are adolescents 'naturally' and inevitably risk-takers or are there other explanations?

Psychologists have put forward a number of theories to explain the so-called risk-taking behaviour in adolescents. There is the sensation-seeking theory (suggesting that adolescents crave excitement), the 'egocentric' theory (suggesting that the young have difficulty in taking anyone's perspective other than their own), the problem behaviour theory (suggesting that risk-taking is a means of winning high status in a group of friends, especially, as far as boys are concerned, in front of girls), the prototype model (young people mimic what they regard as adult behaviour, for example, in smoking and alcohol consumption), and the decision-making model (adolescents who take risks perceive the costs of such behaviour as less than those who don't, and consequently make decisions on the basis of a less favourable cost-benefit calculation).

Most of these explanations are not special to the teenage group. As we know, some people crave excitement throughout their lives. Many do not lose interest in impressing others at least until middle age and often beyond. Calculating the cost of what we do is part of decision-making throughout life, and there is a good evidence that those in their teens have as realistic idea of the dangers of different risks as their parents. For example, Ruth Beyth-Maron, an American psychologist, found extraordinary similarity when she compared nearly 200 young people in their teens with their parents, in how they evaluated the risk involved in six different types of behaviour. There is no very convincing foundation for any of these explanations being special to the teen years. Another more convincing way of looking at the so-called risk-taking at this time of life may be more useful.

Beginners are accident-prone. The 14-month-old making his first wobbly attempts at walking will fall over a good deal more than the confident two-year-old. The heart surgeon undertaking a complicated operation for the first time will have a higher fatality rate than another surgeon with much more experience. They are both doing as much as they can to avoid taking risks and hurting themselves or others. Because they are doing something new, they have to experiment to see what works. The toddler tries to run before he can walk. The heart surgeon may try different approaches to an inaccessible blood vessel he wants to tie off. But it would be silly to suggest that 14-month-olds or heart surgeons are risk-takers. The teen years are the time when young people experience numerous enjoyable but also potentially dangerous situations, driving cars, having sex, drinking alcohol, using illegal drugs, for the first time. Apart from driving lessons, proper preparation and initiation into the skills required to manage these activities is usually hit and miss, to say the least. It is hardly surprising that mistakes, and sometimes mistakes with very serious consequences, are made.

Another reason why teenagers take risks is that their social situation means there are some activities that are difficult to perform except in risky ways. This is particularly true of sex. The fully mature 16-year-old couple who have the opportunity to have full sexual intercourse from time to time (often at unpredictable times) in one of their family homes or at the home of a friend are likely to find it much more difficult to take precautions against pregnancy or infection than a 25-year-old couple who are living together and can plan to have condoms or other means of protection available all the time.

When it comes to risky sporting activities, it is difficult to see how one could justify the idea that it is the period of adolescence in which most risks are taken. Formula One motor racing, motorcycle racing, mountain climbing, cave exploration, scuba diving, parachuting, and hang-gliding, the most dangerous sporting activities in terms of the risk of death, are not teenage pastimes, but engaged in mainly by those in their mid and late twenties.

Now as we shall see later in this chapter, there is one small group of young people in their teens that can be regarded as serious risk-takers and very worrying they are too. This is the group that is suffering from the type of serious antisocial behaviour that persists throughout life and they are further described later in this chapter. When an 18-year-old, who has been impulsive, impetuous, and unable to resist the slightest temptation continuously since early childhood is given the opportunity to drive a car or drink as much alcohol as he wants, or offered drugs, the temptation not only to experiment but to experiment to excess, may well be too much for him. He is showing a life-long disorder. This does not mean that all adolescents are risk-takers, any more than the fact that adolescents suffer from diabetes or asthma means these are adolescent disorders.

It seems then that the reputation adolescents have for risk-taking can only very occasionally be attributed to a 'natural' tendency on the part of this age group to court danger. Their relatively high risk for injury or death can be largely explained on the basis of the fact that they are embarking on what are new activities for them for which they have been poorly prepared or because their social situation makes it difficult for them to undertake some potentially risky activities except in dangerous ways. Just occasionally it is because they are showing a lifelong problem. So adolescents are not 'naturally' risk-takers; they just live in a riskier world than do younger children or older people.

5.6 **Crime and the teens**

There are four common beliefs about crime and the teens. The first, that is only partly accurate, is that the highest rates of offending are found in those in their teen years. There are two main sources of information. The first is the Home Office Youth Lifestyles Survey, 2000. This involved 4848 young people aged between 12 and 30 years who were asked about the numbers of offences they had committed. The commonest ages for admitting to offending were between 18 and 21 years. If, instead of looking at self-reports of offending, one looks at crime statistics collected by the police, one finds that the highest rates are spread between 16 and 20 years, with about the same numbers of 21–24-year-olds found guilty of or cautioned for offences as are 15-year-olds. So the highest rates of offending are spread well beyond the teen years.

The second belief is that most of those in their teens are committing crimes all the time. This belief is totally inaccurate. In fact, the same self-report survey showed that only one in five boys and young men admitted to committing an offence in the previous year. Most of those young people who had offended had only committed one or two offences. A very small minority of young people (2% of the males and less than 1% of the females) had committed nearly half the crimes. The third belief is equally inaccurate. It is that the rate of crime committed by the young goes up all the time. In fact, the percentage of 15–17-year-old boys found guilty or cautioned for an offence in any one year went down from about 7.5% in 1991 to about 6% in 2001, a marked reduction of about 20% from the higher figure. The numbers of girls also went down though to a lesser degree. The fourth belief is that the young are more likely to commit offences than to be the victims of offences. Unfortunately, because the excellent British Crime Survey of victims of crime carried out by the Home Office does not involve questioning of people below the age of 16 years we cannot be sure this is inaccurate, but easily the greatest chance (about 16% in boys and 7% in girls) of being a victim is in the youngest group questioned, the 16–24-year age group. This strongly suggests that those younger than 16 years also have much greater chances of being a victim than of committing an offence.

5.7 **Two types of antisocial behaviour**

It has fairly recently been shown that, among those in their teens, there are two reasonably distinct pathways into offending behaviour. A team of investigators now working at the Institute of Psychiatry, London, led by Terrie Moffitt and Avshalom Caspi, have carried out a study in Dunedin, New Zealand, of a group of people from when they were three years old until their late twenties in the early years of the twenty-first century.

Looking at those who were in trouble because of their antisocial behaviour in adolescence, they found two reasonably distinct groups. The first group showed problems from their very early years, continued during childhood and the teens, and then well into adult life. They called the antisocial behaviour of this group 'Life-Course Persistent', or LCP for short.

The second group only began to show serious antisocial behaviour (especially marked disobedience, stealing, fighting, and general aggressiveness), at some point between round about 10 or 11 years and the end of the teens. They called the antisocial behaviour of this group 'Adolescence-Limited', or AL for short. Here are stories of two boys caught for the same crime, but clearly very different, the first from the LCP group and the second from the AL group.

Keith is 15-years-old. He has been arrested for the fifth time in 12 months. With two other boys he has been caught in a stolen car. Keith can break into most cars in a couple of minutes. Shortly after he was born to his then 17-year-old mother, Keith was taken into care, and fostered for about nine months. At that point, his mother was living in a flat with a man, not Keith's father, five years older than herself, and asked to have him home. Doubtful social workers agreed, and decided to keep a close watch on how he fared. But there were changes in staff in the Social Work Department, Keith's mother moved away, and he was lost to supervision. Around the age of two and a half, his mother was in touch once again with Social Services, and he was admitted to a Day Nursery where he was regarded as overactive and very difficult. At four and a half years he started 'proper school', and soon the teachers were asking for help with him. He was disruptive in class, calling out names and wandering about when he should have been sitting still. At five and a half, his mother said she couldn't cope with him at home any more. She was now living with an unemployed van driver, who couldn't stand Keith and beat him up badly when he didn't do what he was told, which was a good deal of the time. He was re-admitted to a children's home. He has lived in four different places between six years and the present time, the longest being four years in a foster home where eventually his two remarkable foster parents said they could no longer manage him. He has remained in mainstream school, because his mother, of whom he is very fond, and who has continued to keep in touch and occasionally has him home for weekends, has refused to allow him to go to a special school. But he is still only able to read as well as an average seven-year-old, despite a great deal of remedial help. All his friends are in similar trouble to himself. Drink and drugs find their way into the children's home, and two of the older girls are involved in prostitution. Keith will now, almost certainly be sent to a secure unit for young offenders. Follow-up studies suggest that he has about an 85% chance of a long-lasting criminal career once he reaches adulthood.

The second example is a very different boy, though caught by the police for the same type of offence.

Wayne is also 15 years old, and has been picked up breaking into a car with two other boys. He had been celebrating the victory of the Midlands football team he supports with his friends, and they had continued to drink until after midnight. Starting to walk home, they had got bored with the long distance, and one of his friends said he knew how to get into a car. It had taken so long to work the lock that they had been spotted, someone had informed the police and the three, none of whom had ever been arrested before, had been picked up. This is Wayne's first detected offence, though he has been skirting round trouble with the police for the last two years. He has been truanting fairly persistently and has missed a good deal of school. He is a big lad, and, on two occasions, again after drinking, has got involved in fights at football matches, and hurt someone badly enough that they have had to be taken to an Accident and Emergency Department. Wayne's early life was unremarkable. His parents were married and already had a daughter, Janice, aged 2 years, when he was born. His father, also a van driver, has always been in work, and his mother has worked part-time as a shop assistant since Wayne was three years old, so the family has never been hard up. He was a cuddly baby and both his parents have always been fond of him, and have shown a good deal of affection to him. Wayne got on well at his primary school, and made good friends there. He was popular and in the school football team. Trouble began when Wayne moved *to secondary school. It happened that most of his friends went to different schools, and Wayne did not find it easy to make new friends. He did not much like the school, and found it boring. The sports facilities were poor, and the PE teaching staff unenthusiastic and demoralized. At the same time, his mother got depressed and irritable. Though the two children do not know this, she had become aware that her husband has formed another relationship. Now he is out of the house much more. Janice has a boyfriend, and is doing so well at school that she is on track to go to the University. After the police and probation department had made enquiries and discovered Wayne's poor school attendance, he was charged and put on probation. Wayne has a lot going for him. The probation officer found a club with a football team for him. He started going out with a girl and she told him she would give him up if he got into trouble again. The school began to keep a much closer eye on his attendance. He started to get interested in the Design and Technology classes and discovered he was good on computers. With his background, Wayne has less than a 10% chance of developing persistent criminal behaviour as an adult, though he will probably always be more of a risk-taker than most people.*

Keith and Wayne have both been convicted of the same offence, but it is clear that the circumstances leading up to the two offences are different and that the outlook for the two of them is dramatically different.

5.8 Life-course persistent (LCP) antisocial behaviour

This is a very serious problem both for the individual and for society. It occurs around 10 times more often in boys than in girls. Fortunately, there are far fewer boys with this type of difficulty than there are with AL antisocial behaviour, though the amount of trouble they cause to themselves and to the neighbourhoods in which they live is no greater. More than half the offences committed by the teenage population is carried out by this group who come from only one in twenty of the age group. How does LCP antisocial behaviour show itself?

Problems may begin in the first few weeks or months of life when the baby may be restless, difficult to settle, and slow to develop a regular pattern of eating and sleeping. The baby is showing personality or temperamental features that make him difficult to manage. The family into which this difficult baby is born is usually under stress for one reason or another. Usually, though not always, the home is unsettled and sometimes, as in the case of Keith whose life I described earlier in this chapter, very unsettled. Perhaps because it seems an easy way out or perhaps because this is the way the parents themselves were brought up and they know no other way, the child is likely to be reared in the manner described in Chapter 3 as 'authoritarian', lacking in early 'attunement', with little sensitivity to the emotional needs of the child and harsh punishment. The man in the family is likely to resort to physical violence when faced with disagreement with another family member, whether this shows itself, for example, as a toddler's disobedience or a partner's unwillingness to have sex.

Often because they are in financial difficulties or living in overcrowded circumstances, parents may not have the time to take much interest in the child's feelings or point of view. By two or three years of life the child with LCP antisocial behaviour (usually but not always a boy, for this pattern is about 10 times more common in boys) is overactive, distractible, and difficult to manage. Such children often show hyperactivity as toddlers and young children. They cannot sit at table for more than a minute or two. Their attention span is short, and they cannot look at a book or attempt a jigsaw or colour in pictures for more than a few moments. Although he may be mesmerized by television or a video and watch it for hours on end, a hyperactive child will not be able to concentrate nor understand much of what is happening on the screen.

The boy's language may be slow to develop and he may be thought to be deaf. At playgroup or nursery school, the child with this type of antisocial behaviour will be disruptive and difficult. The teacher is likely to complain to the mother about the child's behaviour, and other parents may ask for the child to be removed. He may well be sent to a clinic and diagnosed as showing ADHD or 'attention deficit hyperactivity disorder'. Once the child enters infant school, other problems emerge. There are likely to be difficulties in learning to read, perhaps because the child cannot seem to discriminate between the different letter shapes, or because he cannot concentrate long enough to make the connection between letters and sounds. Difficulties in reading may be part of a more general language problem.

The child may now begin to show behaviour arising from his frustration at not being able to keep up with other children, and perhaps also because he is experiencing rejection. At home, his parents will be finding it increasingly difficult to avoid being constantly angry and hostile to him because of his disobedience and irritating behaviour. At school, few, if any children will want to play with him because he is seen to cause trouble and may get them into trouble. In the neighbourhood, he may well be regarded as a pest, breaking windows, hitting other children, and spoiling their games. The rejection he experiences may lead to further bad behaviour, often escalating at this point into violence. He may be excluded from school.

By now, as he moves into his teens, all or most of his friends will also be in trouble. He will be seen as a risk-taker, and indeed he certainly is. He will be committing offences, perhaps breaking into cars, getting into fights, stealing from shops. At some point, he will be charged and, after various attempts have been made to intervene without removing him from the community, he will be sent to an institution for young offenders. There he will meet older, professional criminals who will socialize him into a criminal culture, giving him a new language and skills to survive by breaking the law. (All the evidence suggests that, far from acting as a deterrent, custodial sentences increase the likelihood of further offending.) Once discharged, the antisocial skills he has learned may enable him, by now an adult, to keep out of an institution for young offenders or prison for a few months or years, but eventually he will be charged with a more serious offence and receive a long custodial sentence. By this point, it is likely that he will show various personality characteristics that make it difficult for him to hold a job and get on with other people. He is probably suspicious, sensitive, and easily upset. He has the sense of being constantly 'got at' and victimized. It will not be easy for him to make new friends. His life once he reaches middle age is less predictable, because although numerous follow-up studies have charted the career of such children from infancy to early adulthood, so far they have stopped short before the individuals concerned have reached their forties.

Life-course persistent antisocial behaviour is not an adolescent disorder, any more than are physical conditions like cerebral palsy or spina bifida that may be present in the teens. All these start in infancy and present problems throughout life. Young people with chronic physical problems may have particular difficulties in adolescence, perhaps because, for the first time, they have sexual feelings no one explains to them, or because they are more often left out or rejected by their friends, but no one would dream of calling cerebral palsy or spina bifida adolescent disorders.

Of course, the course of events is not always as dismal as the above account makes it sound. Further, it is important to stress that most boys who show hyperactivity or ADHD are not also seriously disobedient and aggressive, and do not show this pattern of antisocial behaviour. Especially if their parents are reasonably warm and accepting of them, while laying down clear limits to what is and is not permitted, most children with ADHD have a much better outlook. Forbearing teachers who understand that children with ADHD are 'different', and manage to provide structure in the classroom for them can also make a great difference. Most go on to become law-abiding citizens, though perhaps they may choose to follow occupations such as gardener, tour guide, community nurse, travelling salesman, or politician that accommodate their needs for movement and constant stimulation. But some children with ADHD do also go on to show this persistent type of antisocial behaviour.

5.9 Why do children develop life-course persistent antisocial behaviour?

Many readers might think, in view of my description of the typical family from which they come, this is an unnecessary question. But, in fact, most children who come from the sorts of families I have described, although they are at greater risk than others of having persistent antisocial behaviour, go through life without running into such terrible trouble. What is different about those who are less fortunate?

The most striking difference is that, from an early age, there are many signs that they have at least some degree of brain dysfunction. From at least the age of three years, they have an unusual number of abnormalities of their nervous system, such as clumsiness, squints, unequal reflexes, and jerky movements of their eyes. Their language delay and personality difficulties probably also arise from the fact that their brains are built differently from others. When children with these neurological abnormalities are born into families living in adverse circumstances, with parents who are having difficulty coping with life and are reacting aggressively themselves, the risks of life-continuous antisocial behaviour are high.

These neurological abnormalities and other signs of brain dysfunction are as important as the family problems. When girls show them, they are just as likely to develop long-lasting antisocial behaviour as are boys. But many fewer girls have such neurological abnormalities. This difference between the sexes in their frequency of brain dysfunction goes far, perhaps all the way, to explain why girls are so much less likely to show this pattern of lifelong behaviour than are boys.

Why then does the brain dysfunction occur? There is no good evidence that abnormalities in the birth or at the time of delivery are significant. But there are many indications that the dysfunction is at least partly inherited. Many, though by no means all children with lifelong antisocial behaviour begin life showing marked hyperactivity. Studies of twins carried out by Florence Levy in Australia point very strongly to the importance of genes in ADHD. DNA investigations have established the genetic basis of at least some cases of ADHD. Studies of twins also point strongly to the importance of genetic influences in explaining temperamental differences between children.

Many people find it difficult to accept that genes affect the different ways children behave in their early years. But most parents with more than one child will recognize that their children have been different from the first few days of life. They will not feel happy about putting this down to the fact they have brought up their children differently. If this is true of one's own children, why should it not be so for those of other people?

It is also possible that some degree of brain dysfunction comes about because of the difficult circumstances in which such children are brought up. There is evidence that from the early days of life, boys are reared differently from girls; their mothers talk to them less and are less sensitive to their moods and feelings. They are more often encouraged to be assertive, indeed aggressive. Such differences are bound to affect the way the brain works to some degree. Inadequate nutrition in the first few months of life, a problem more likely to occur in disadvantaged families in which children are neglected, also affects brain function. Genes are therefore not the only influence to cause brain dysfunction.

5.10 **What parents can do to prevent life-course persistent antisocial problems**

Recognizing the individuality of babies and young children. As seen in Chapter 3, the most successful forms of parenting are those that involve listening to children and responding to their views and feelings. As these are different from baby to baby and from child to child, this is not a task about which one can generalize. All the same, it is clear that children who are impulsive, overactive, and distractible need much clearer, firmer boundaries set for them than children who do not show these personality features.

Most, though by no means all parents who have children with persistent antisocial behaviour will say they recognized they were 'different' from the first few months of life and certainly from the first year or two. They will have been quite unusually restless and difficult to manage, as well as slow to learn. As they move into their second and third year it is clear that they are unusually disobedient and impulsive.

Providing firm structure with warmth and acceptance is especially difficult with these children, but it is also especially important. Many parents discover they have to be really clear and firm about the boundaries for behaviour they set their children. Those who do not make this discovery run into serious problems. Authoritative methods of parenting, as described in Chapter 3, are the most effective, but they are hard to deliver because such children have difficulties communicating their needs in an acceptable way.

Maintaining good contact with day care and school. It is very easy for parents and teachers to be at cross purposes where these children are concerned. Their disruptive behaviour makes teachers complain that parents are not providing proper discipline. Parents may think that teachers are 'picking on' their children for bad behaviour or don't understand them. The better the communication between parents, day-care workers, and teachers the fewer misunderstandings will occur. Looking after these children is hard enough without getting into a situation of mutual blame and recrimination. Parents and teachers need all the help they can get from each other.

Harm limitation. As children with life-continuous antisocial behaviour move into their teen years, it is likely they will be in serious trouble with the police, beginning to use drugs, truanting, or dropping out of school altogether. Parents will often feel stigmatized by other parents and teachers who point the finger at them for not being able to control their children. It is only too easy for parents in this situation to feel helpless and powerless. Once again they need all the help and support they can get. This is easier if they are able to avoid being defensive and work together with teachers, social workers, the police, and others involved in crime detection and the provision of services. But they do also often need to act as advocates for their children who, by this age, because of their reputations, may be stigmatized and blamed for misdemeanours they haven't committed. They also need to find some enjoyable activities for themselves outside the home so that they are not completely taken up with being parents of very difficult children.

5.11 **What those in authority can do about persistent antisocial behaviour**

Reducing the number of families under financial, housing, and other stress. As I pointed out in Chapter 3, it is a great deal easier for parents to respond sensitively to a child's temperament and individuality if they are living in comfortable accommodation, with enough money not to worry where the next meal is coming from, with a garden at the back, and a park up the road.

Early help and support for parents. Parenting classes that provide information to parents about the most effective methods for providing structure while remaining warm and accepting of their children have been evaluated and shown to work. There are a number of initiatives along these lines, such as the Positive Parenting Programmes developed by Matt Sanders in Queensland, Australia, and by Caroline Webster-Stratton in the United States, that have been shown to work. Parents are given practical advice and helped to achieve positive, firm techniques that do not involve the use of physical punishment. Health visitors, those who work in crèches, day nurseries, and other types of early child care need training in recognizing restless, impulsive, disruptive, and unusually disobedient children, so that they can put parents in touch with those running such programmes or press for them to be developed in the areas in which they work.

Intervention in primary schools. Once such children reach their teen years they are increasingly difficult to help, so that intervention in primary school is crucial. The provision of appropriate remedial help to ensure basic literacy skills are obtained, behaviour support plans that take into account the child's need for structure and continuous warm care, withdrawal units with high staff–child ratios, and a curriculum that improves the child's self-esteem rather than make him feel even more inadequate are all likely to be helpful.

Interventions in secondary schools. These are discussed in some detail in Chapter 9. As with primary schools, the availability of special remedial teaching, the use of behaviour support plans, and the development of withdrawal units have all been found to be helpful.

Finding the balance between helping the individual and protecting the community. The first principle must surely be to avoid making matters worse than they already are. It is now well established that putting young, seriously antisocial male teenagers together in any sort of group care, whether these be boot camps, units for secure offenders, or large children's homes, increases the likelihood the boy or young man will offend again. Such institutions are too often places where young people learn new types of antisocial behaviour and are more often brutalizing than humanizing. It should be added that some youth offender institutions have dedicated, skilled staff who make a real difference to the sense of worth and self-esteem of those in their care. But too often, once boys or young men return to the community, they re-offend, perhaps partly because of the lack of after-care.

But communities do have to be protected from the impact of young people who commit dozens and sometimes hundreds of offences. The most effective or perhaps one should say the least ineffective methods appear to be highly expensive methods, involving keeping the child at home or in treatment foster care. The freedom of the young person is limited, but they and their families are provided with a whole range of interventions by one or two highly trained professionals. In the United States, Scott Henggeler, in the University of South Carolina, has pioneered what he and his colleagues call multi-system family therapy. Individual, well-trained and well-supervised professionals take on families in which young people in their early teens with appalling records of repeated violent offences, out of school, on drugs, from homes mainly headed by unemployed, depressed, lone mothers. Working with the families, gradually trying to empower family members by successfully helping to tackle their life problems one at a time, they achieve better results than psychiatric hospitalisation, or other forms of group care at no greater cost. Until very recently, anyone taking a hard look at the effectiveness of methods of intervening successfully with life-continuous antisocial behaviour would have to admit there was virtually no encouraging information. That situation is now changing. But, of course, if it were possible by a programme of improved parenting of children in their early years, to prevent children from developing such serious behaviour in their teen years that would be far preferable.

Collecting better information. One of the most important ways in which the issue of violence among young people could be tackled is by extending the age of the population, surveyed in the British Crime Survey mentioned earlier, downwards below 16 years at least to 10 years, the current age of criminal responsibility. The 10–16-year-olds are among the most vulnerable groups in society, and it is very disappointing that we do not collect information that would allow us to establish more precisely the extent to which they are victims as well as trends in the prevalence of violent acts over time.

It should be said that governments are now increasingly aware of the need for early intervention if this type of antisocial behaviour is to be reduced. The UK programmes such as SureStart for preschool children and their families and On Track for primary-aged children involve work in disadvantaged areas of the country using all of the approaches I have described. The problem is that, although these programmes have been generously resourced, many remain under-funded, only supported in the short-term, and not universally available to the disadvantaged in all areas.

5.12 Adolescence-limited (AL) antisocial behaviour

This type of offending behaviour is shown by a much larger number of young people in their teens, perhaps one in four, compared to one in twenty of the lifelong persistent type. Those with temporary antisocial behaviour become markedly disobedient at some time in their early teens or just before, and they get into trouble outside the home. Indeed in this respect, they do resemble the stereotype of the caricature of the Harry Enfield nightmare teenagers who, I suggested in Chapter 1, are unfairly portrayed on television and in the press as typical of the whole of the teen generation. I am not talking here of young people (unconventional to adults, but conventional in their peer group), who wear what to older people appear to be outrageous clothes, nose-rings or tongue-studs or belly metal, amazing hairstyles and colours, or get involved in struggles with the rules their parents try to lay down.

The group with temporary antisocial behaviour who contribute to the crime statistics have more serious problems. First, they are much more severely disobedient, especially as far as obeying rules set by their parents. As well as smoking and drinking heavily, they are likely to get involved with illegal drugs, showing not just occasional but regular use. They may sometimes sell drugs, though usually only to friends and acquaintances. They may get into fights with others of their age. In school, this takes the form of bullying. Out of school, they are quite likely to have been drinking when they become violent. They may be involved in damaging property, throwing bricks through windows, twisting off wing mirrors, scratching the metalwork of cars, or damaging them in other ways. Stealing car radios or wheel hubs, shoplifting, nicking mobile phones, or taking money from home are other common offences. More seriously they may get involved in burglary, breaking and entering homes and stealing what they can readily take away.

Those in their teens who show temporary antisocial behaviour are different from lifelong offenders in that their offences, though often quite serious, begin in the teens, end no later than the mid-twenties and often go on for only a few months or a couple of years. But they are different in many other ways. Especially as far as severe disobedience and using drugs are concerned, they are just as likely to be girls as well as boys. The other types of offence, especially those involving stealing and physically aggressive behaviour, are more likely to be committed by boys, but it is now common for girls to be involved in this behaviour too. Temporary offenders usually do not commit very large numbers of crimes or be involved in the most serious crimes. They are unlikely to injure other people seriously. Although there are many times, perhaps 10 times more temporary than there are LCP offenders, because those with lifelong problems commit crimes so much more frequently, they are responsible for about as many crimes.

5.13 Why does 'teen-temporary' antisocial behaviour occur?

The Maturity Gap: The rate of crime overall and, in particular, the age when criminal activity peaks, has much to do with the position of young people in their mid to late teens and early twenties in our society. Over the last fifty years, the age when young people become financially and emotionally independent has extended into the late teens and early twenties. At the same time, the peak age for offending has moved from the early teens to the late teens. It is clear that if young people are not allowed to take responsibility, they will have a greater tendency to behaving irresponsibly.

Personal reasons: These young people have not, in general, been very different in their personalities and in many other ways from their contemporaries in childhood up to their early teens. They may have been a little more outgoing, a bit more adventurous, and not have done quite as well in school, but the differences are small. Basically these have been 'normal' children, not standing out as remarkable in any way.

On the other hand, their families are often different. They may have younger parents and are more likely to be living with lone parents. Other family members, especially their parents, may have been involved in antisocial behaviour and have police records themselves. One or both parents may have mental health problems, usually a tendency to become depressed or anxious. Arguments between parents especially over money, over other relationships, and about bringing up the children are common. The boy or girl with temporary antisocial behaviour is often living in a family in difficult financial circumstances, with one or both parents unemployed on a long-term basis. All this may mean that parents are not able to keep an eye on what their children are doing. The sort of supervision one would expect 9–13-year-old children to respond to is lacking.

There are many young people living in such circumstances, but only some of these are triggered into showing temporary antisocial behaviour. The triggers are well known. Home may suddenly become a much more depressing place. The parents may split up or a lone mother, with whom the child has developed a close relationship, may begin an intimate friendship with a new partner with whom the child does not get on. The feelings of rejection may lead to arguments so that all the young person wants to do is to get out of the house or flat. A new baby with a new partner may take up all the attention with little left for a teenager who feels pushed out.

All of this young people may be able to cope with, if school is going well and they have good friends in the neighbourhood who are not in trouble themselves. But if to add to their troubles at home, the young person starts to irritate and be irritated by a particular teacher, begins to find a number of subjects difficult or boring, or is the butt of teasing from others in the class, then the behaviour that may get the individual into serious trouble is quite likely to occur.

This is more likely to happen if the child begins to mix with others who have already got into trouble with the police for the sorts of behaviour I have described. This may happen to boys because an older brother or sister is in such a group. Girls who mature early are especially at risk. Their physical appearance may mean they get involved with older teenagers, and be expected to behave in ways they cannot cope with emotionally. Early sexual experience for which they are poorly prepared and regular drug use may follow. In neighbourhoods with unusually high delinquency rates, such as those council estates where violence and drug problems are endemic, it is much more likely that young people with personal stresses at home or at school will become involved in temporary antisocial behaviour.

5.14 **What parents can do about temporary behaviour problems**

The fact that young people who get involved in antisocial behaviour for the first time in their teen years are normal in so many ways and have a pretty good outlook is encouraging news for parents and teachers who would like to see such behaviour occur less frequently. What can they do? In Chapter 3, I have suggested ways parents can help to prevent difficult behaviour from occurring in the first place. It is clearly more satisfactory as well as easier to prevent antisocial behaviour than to deal with it once it has started. The key to success in helping those in their teens to stay out of trouble is the establishment of sensitivity to the child's needs early on in life, followed by authoritative parenting (as described in Chapter 3), in middle childhood and the early teens.

Most parents, even those living in disadvantaged circumstances, manage to achieve this. They may have had harsh, punitive parents themselves in their own childhood, but they are less likely than their parents to use such methods to bring up their own children in this way. They are more likely to enter into negotiations with their children over disagreements than were their own parents and less likely just to lay down the law. They are more likely to treat their own children as individuals with personalities of their own than to assume that all children are born the same. So when there are the sorts of stresses in the family that might trigger antisocial behaviour, they are also more likely to be sensitive to how their teenage children are feeling, to find the time to listen to them, and to give them the attention they need. In return, their teenage children are likely to respect them more and to be more helpful when their parents are themselves going through a difficult time.

When Brian, who had been living alone on a rough council estate with his single mother since he was 6, turned 15 years, she began a friendship with a divorced man older than herself at the shop where she worked as an assistant and where he was the manager. She had avoided such relationships before because she had not wanted Brian to feel pushed out. Now he had reached his mid-teens she felt safer to do so and indeed had become worried how she would cope when Brian made more of an independent life for himself. But Brian was not one little bit happy about his mother's friend. He made derogatory remarks about the man after he had met him and tried to talk his mother into giving up her job and going to work elsewhere. His mother was put out, but decided she was fond of this man and was not going to be put off by her son. All the same, she became much more discreet about seeing him and did not bring him home again. She made more time for Brian and, if anything, tried to make sure the two of them did more things together rather than less. After a time, Brian found himself a girlfriend and, because he told his mother most things, he talked to her about this girl. In a light-hearted way, his mother then began to make comparisons with her own relationship and became more open about it. Brian began to suggest his mother brought her friend home, but his mother decided this might bring back the feelings of jealousy again. Eventually, Brian became much less involved in his mother's life. The two were able to separate, though if his mother had not been able to take her son's feelings into account, he might well have become involved in some of the quite serious antisocial activities going on in the council estate where they lived.

5.15 How society can make it easier for teens at risk of AL antisocial behaviour to keep out of trouble

Unfortunately, the first reaction of any government faced with public concern about what are, as we have seen, misperceptions of rising rates of crime, is likely to be punitive. This is the case at the time of writing in the autumn of 2003 when, in England and Wales, the government proposes to introduce an Antisocial Behaviour Bill aimed chiefly at the young. Permission to the police to break up groups of two or more children, the introduction of child curfews, fixed fines exacted by head teachers for absence from school, and heavy penalties for parents when children are caught in possession of drugs, are unlikely to do more to cut crime than similar punitive measures introduced in the past. Whenever punitive measures are scientifically evaluated, they turn out to be ineffective deterrents.

Reducing the stress on families. All measures that ensure that families with teenage children have enough money to live on and decent living conditions will reduce offending behaviour. This can only happen when there is economic stability providing employment opportunities for both men and women who are sufficiently educated to take advantage of them. With the expanding population, sufficient decent housing with enough space for those in their teens to have at least some privacy, can only become available if housing policy is changed both to increase the number of housing units and to make housing more affordable for families with teenage children. This is especially true for those whose parents are working in relatively low-paid public service occupations such as nursing and teaching in places where housing is expensive.

Financial support for temporary or more permanent lone parenthood. Lone parenthood is usually a temporary phase. Most lone parents are separated or divorced women who find other partners within months or years. Teens in lone parent families, temporary though they may be, are especially liable to become involved in antisocial behaviour. But this does not mean that a reduction in the number of lone parent families would result in reduction in antisocial behaviour. Warring, argumentative couples are also liable to have children who commit crimes. Measures that reduce domestic arguments and especially domestic violence are likely to have an impact on the rate of teenage offending behaviour whether or not they prevent the break-down of marriages or cohabitations. These will include any encouragement or help that society can provide to parents to enable them to sort out their conflicts amicably. Children who are brought up by parents who have themselves been reared using authoritative methods, as described in Chapter 3, will have more highly developed negotiating skills they can then use when they become parents themselves. Effective education of parents at risk of providing harsh and insensitive child-rearing in the use of authoritative methods could achieve such a result, as could parenting education along similar lines in schools.

Absent fathers are not in themselves, as is often suggested, necessarily a cause of antisocial behaviour. Indeed the disappearance of a father from a family may result in breaking a cycle of violence. But the presence of two parents and of a law-abiding, caring male role model reduces the stress on families and thus the likelihood of antisocial behaviour in teenage children. All measures that promote the involvement of fathers, such as statutory paternity leave and family-friendly work places that accept the need for fathers to spend time with their families, will reduce the likelihood of boys becoming involved in antisocial behaviour.

Making school relevant to the needs of the young people who attend is a tremendous challenge. Ways in which many schools are meeting this challenge are described in Chapter 9. Here it just needs pointing out that boredom at school is a major reason for truancy, which, in itself, is a pathway to many other forms of antisocial behaviour.

Improving leisure facilities, discussed in more detail in Chapter 10, will also have the effect of diverting young people from behaving antisocially. The availability of well-run sporting and other non-academic activities has been shown to reduce the rate of delinquent behaviour in neighbourhoods with high crime rates.

Effective neighbourhood policing is one of a variety of measures needed to make crime more difficult. If there is a high risk that crime will be detected, it is much less likely to occur. *The successful promotion of community support systems,* especially on those estates where racial tensions are high, many young people are unemployed, and drug use is endemic, will result in neighbours being more willing to contact the police or to take other deterrent action if they suspect a group of young people is about to commit a crime.

Improving the security of personal and public property will have a similar effect. If the cars that the two boys, Wayne and Keith, who broke into them, had been alarmed or fitted with steering wheel locks, attempts would not have been made to steal them. Making antisocial behaviour more difficult to carry out successfully is one of the most effective means of prevention. This does not solve the underlying problems of frustration, boredom, disappointment, and depression, but it makes it more likely that these can be addressed in a more appropriate manner.

Incidentally, although I have discussed the importance of measures such as effective policing, improving security of personal property, and fostering a sense of community identity in relation to temporary offending behaviour, they are, of course, of equal importance in preventing crimes committed by LCP offenders. Although these types of offenders may be different, the offences they commit are similar. Indeed, as I suggested earlier in this chapter, the temporary offender may be led into crime by contact with the persistent offender who has, by the teens, become an expert in crime and evasion.

Promoting emotional maturity and social skills before and in the early stages of puberty is helpful for all young people but especially necessary for those girls who mature physically early. Such girls are at risk for mixing with older boys and girls and becoming involved in sexual behaviour before they are emotionally ready for such experiences. As discussed in more detail in Chapter 6, sex education in primary school aiming not just to help children learn about the physical aspects of sex and its consequences, but also about the handling of emotional relationships does not result in earlier involvement in sexual activity and enables the young person to deal with these issues with greater awareness and sensitivity.

Tackling the acceptance of violence as a normal means of conflict resolution. Violence is commonly defined as behaviour by people against people liable to cause physical or psychological harm. A significant amount of antisocial behaviour during the teen years involves violence of one sort or another. Fighting, bullying, mugging, and other forms of street violence all fall into this category. But not all violence is physical. Humiliation, merciless teasing, sarcasm, socially isolating, and relentless criticism are all forms of violence likely to cause psychological harm.

Society is inconsistent in its attitudes to violence. While on the one hand most forms of violence are condemned, others are condoned or even valued. In the House of Commons, at the highest level in the land, politicians seek to make their points not only by logical means, but by humiliating those on the opposite side. Derisive, mocking laughter follows when a government minister appears to fail to make a case adequately. The use of sarcasm by teachers as a means of 'putting down' children is commonly used in our classrooms. Physical punishment, even severe physical punishment of children by parents remains legal and is still widely thought of as acceptable. Only recently, after much campaigning, has domestic violence been taken seriously by the police, magistrates, and the public.

From the early years, male macho violence is valued and its absence taken as evidence of lack of masculinity. There is now widespread concern at the amount of bullying that goes on in school, but the attitude that 'boys will be boys' and that there is nothing society can or indeed should do about bullying remains prevalent. Much antisocial behaviour involves violence that goes beyond, but not far beyond behaviour that is widely acceptable. To reduce the level of antisocial behaviour there needs to be a change in public attitudes to violence and a much lower threshold for the acceptability of violence as a means of resolving conflict.

Reducing exposure of the population to violence-inducing images. There are increasing amounts of physical violence shown on television and available on video. On average there are six murders an hour on terrestrial television, the number having doubled over the last 10 years of the twentieth century. Violent computer games are increasing in popularity. There is evidence that boys who watch more violent television programmes than others are also more likely to show violence in real life. In itself, this would not demonstrate convincingly that exposure to violent images is involved in causing violence. It could just be that violent boys are attracted to watch more violent programmes. But there is strong additional evidence from studies of boys from childhood to adolescence that suggests that, even after taking into account their earlier level of violence, boys who have watched a good deal of violent television before puberty are more violent in real life in their teen years than those who have been exposed to fewer violent images in their childhood.

Research carried out by the British Board of Film Classification (BBFC) with a nationally representative sample, suggested that the catogories of 'U/PG', '12' and '15' allowed too much violence to be shown. The national survey results supported the '18' guidelines as about right. Nevertheless, perhaps in response to the results with other, less representative samples, the BBFC is taking an increasingly relaxed attitude to violence in classification of films and videos at the '18' level, which many poorly supervised young people in their earlier teens are bound to see. Although there is no evidence that such exposure plays more than a minor part in causing violent behaviour, other factors, such as the presence of violent role models in the family being more important, a tougher attitude to classification of violent images on film, television, and in computer games could be expected to lead to a reduction in violence in real life. The desensitization to violence that follows exposure to violent images is especially likely to occur in vulnerable young people, who are already impulsive, sensation-seeking, and living in emotionally disturbing circumstances.

Providing drop-in clinics for teenagers under stress. When faced with stressful situations such as a crisis at home, a fear of pregnancy, concern over the experience of homosexual feelings, or being the target of racist attacks in the neighbourhood, many young people will find sufficient support from their families and friends to see them through difficult times. But others need a place to turn where they can receive advice, information, and emotional support. For some, their family doctor, practice nurse, or practice counsellor can play this role and some practices have special clinics for young people. As we shall see in Chapter 6, where advice on contraception and pregnancy is discussed, if they attend the same practice as their parents, some young people are worried that what they say to their family doctor will not be treated as confidential. One way of dealing with this is to improve the training of doctors, nurses, and practice receptionists so that they can be reassuring about confidentiality. Drop-in clinics at schools and colleges of further education, described further in Chapter 6, can also provide accessible and confidential advice given by nurses and counsellors who have been trained to respond to the predicaments of young people. If such clinics deal not just with emotional problems, but with a range of health problems, it will be easier for young people to attend them without feeling embarrassed or stigmatized.

Developing a new approach to drugs and alcohol. Much crime in the teens is linked to the sale and use of illegal drugs and excessive consumption of alcohol. As I suggest in Chapter 7, there is very little likelihood that there will be a change in such behaviour by those in their teens if it does not occur in the rest of the adult population. And this is most unlikely to happen unless, as I suggest in the later chapter there are changes both in the law on drugs and in public attitudes to the violence linked to both drugs and alcohol.

Treating children as children and those in their teens as young, though inexperienced adults. I have suggested that children with persistent antisocial behaviour show behaviour in their very early years that responds much better to the setting of firmer boundaries than is the case with most children. In contrast, once they enter the teen years, the rate of temporary antisocial behaviour is likely to be reduced if young people are provided with greater levels of responsibility, alternative leisure opportunities, and more relevant education. Though there may be no difference in the community responses required, very different family and psychological approaches are needed to tackle the two different sorts of problematic behaviour. Parents need more authority and respect if they are to tackle the first type of difficulty; they need to be able to consult with and allow their teenage children greater autonomy if temporary offending is to be prevented. This is particularly important as young people move into their mid-to-late teens and into their early twenties; tackling the 'maturity gap' I mentioned earlier in this chapter, by giving those of this age as much independence and responsibility for choices affecting them as possible.

In addition, the juvenile justice system should be in line with the differences between children before puberty and those who have reached adult levels of understanding. Thus, for example, as I suggest in Chapter 11, it would be a step in the right direction if the age of criminal responsibility in the UK were raised from 10 years, as it is at present, to 14 years as it is in most other European countries. Similarly, it would be helpful if court procedures affirmed parental responsibility until the early to mid-teens, but acknowledged that, after that age, however much they might wish to, there is often a limit to what parents can do to enforce rules on their children.

This proposal will rightly raise concerns among people who would be worried about exposing young people in their mid-teens to the United Kingdom adult justice system with its almost exclusive emphasis on punitive approaches to crime. Bringing young people in their mid-teens into the adult justice system needs to wait until the system, at least for those convicted of crimes under the age of twenty five years, has become much more strongly rehabilitational in its approach. This needs to happen as a matter of urgency.

Chapter 6

Sex: same hormones, different lives

6.1 Introduction

Myths, or widely held inaccurate ideas about sex and the teens, are common in the adult world, so that much discussion is poorly informed.

What are these myths? First, is the idea that the physical changes of puberty begin in the teens. In fact, they begin well before this. Indeed they begin well before these physical changes are visible. Another myth is that sexual development is beginning earlier these days than it did even 20 years ago. The evidence for this is weak or non-existent. A third myth is those in their teens have extraordinarily high levels of sex hormones, and that these gradually decline in the twenties. Finally, there is a widespread and mistaken notion that all those in their teens are, or at least would like to be, highly promiscuous in their sexual behaviour.

These myths are unhelpful. What the adult world surely needs to do is to prepare children for sexual development and experience, protect them against premature sexualization, and to empower young people, once they choose to do so, to enter into sexual relationships caringly, enjoyably, and safely.

The truth is less dramatic than the myths, and, in any case, perhaps the most important fact for the adult world to understand about sex in the teens is the diversity of physical development, sexual orientation, interest in sex, and sexual behaviour. In this chapter, I shall explore these issues and then suggest ways in which the adult world might better prepare, protect, and finally empower the young in their sexual lives.

6.2 Diversity of sex and relationships in the two worlds of adolescence

Mary is 17 years old. She lives with her parents in a three bedroom house on the outskirts of a small town in the Home Counties. The family income is low, only just above the poverty line, as her father has a low paid job as a shop assistant in a local electrical shop. However, she and her younger brother have enjoyed great stability and affection in their lives.

From the age of five when she went to infant school, Mary has had the same best friend, a girl she met on her very first day. She also mixed with a wider group of girls, many of whom transferred with her, as did her best friend, into the local comprehensive school at the age of 11 years. Until they were 14 or 15 years old, none of these girls mixed much with boys, although many of them, like Mary, had brothers in their families.

From about the age of 13 years, shortly after her first period, Mary has had powerful, intense, sexual fantasies. Before these began, she had a 'crush' on a female teacher, but her fantasies about this teacher were not strictly speaking sexual, involving just going on holiday with her, having long talks, and cuddling. At 13 years though, she began to have exciting fantasies about sexual play with a boy in the next form up, a young man much admired by her girlfriends for his good looks and general sociability. All her friends thought he was smashing looking, and they used to joke about kidnapping him and taking him off to one of their homes and what they would do to him there. Mary did not make much of a contribution to this fantasy chat, though she joined in the giggling that went with it. Instead, in the privacy of her bedroom, she imagined long sessions of petting, ending in intercourse with him. During one of these fantasies she experienced a spontaneous orgasm, and then started to masturbate herself to orgasm once or twice a week. She did not tell anybody about these fantasies or her masturbation, of which she was deeply ashamed, even though she had been told at school that masturbation was 'normal'. The subject of her fantasies changed from time to time, usually involving boys in higher classes, but once a young male teacher. She never attempted to have a relationship with any of the boys or men in her fantasies, and they never made any advances to her.

When she turned sixteen, Charles, the brother of one of her friends, whom she had met at her friend's house, began to take an interest in her and asked if she would go with him to a party. She liked the look of him, and agreed. He seemed a gentle, caring young man, a couple of years older than she. They began to go out together regularly, to the cinema, parties, and occasionally a club. Her parents insisted she was home at midnight, and she had no problem with this rule, though occasionally she would ask for an extension and this would be granted. Charles's mother is a single parent, his father having left home when Charles was twelve. But, after a difficult time, his mother has recovered from her depression, and his father is in touch with him, and takes an interest in his life. The two go out together once a fortnight or so.

Mary and Charles are fond of each other. They have similar interests. He is taking 'A' levels and she her GCSEs. They discuss their work, their teachers, their friends, and enjoy gossiping about who is going out with who, who is being dumped, and so on. They like the same sort of music.

A physical relationship began about a month after they started to go out together. With her parents downstairs, they would kiss and cuddle in her bedroom while they were ostensibly listening to music. Soon, Charles wanted to go further, tried to caress her breasts and stroke her thighs. He was quite persistent. She knew from the experience of her fantasies, that if she let him do this she would be unable to stop him from having intercourse with her and she did not know whether she wanted this. So far, for about a year, she has held him off. He sometimes has an orgasm while they are kissing and she doesn't like this, but cannot bring herself to tell him. She wants to have a full sexual relationship with him as she does in her masturbatory fantasies, but something holds her back. She has discussed what to do with her best friend who counsels caution. Her friend was dropped by her long-standing boyfriend after she had sex with him a few times. She wants to talk with other people, perhaps including her mother, but she cannot bring herself to do so.

Mary is distressed, but she does have choice. If she decides to 'go all the way', she knows she will first go to the doctor and get birth control advice. She is in control of the situation. But Charles is also in control of what happens next. He can cope with his frustration by dropping Mary and going out with one of the group who, he knows, takes a more relaxed attitude to sex. But he is very fond of Mary and does not really want to do this. He does not want to hurt her, but he desperately wants sex with her. The possibility fills his mind. He cannot concentrate on his schoolwork. So both these young people have choices.

Jane is also 17 years old, and is an only child. She lives in a flat on a council estate about half a mile from Mary. Her father left home when she was a baby. Since that time her mother has lived with three men, the relationships lasting between a month and four years. At present her mother is without a partner. The shortest relationship was the last, and occurred when Jane was twelve. Her mother's partner attempted to have sex with Jane, who promptly told her mother. He was told to get out and Jane's mother has not lived with another man since. However before that time, Jane saw her mother engaged in many flirtatious relationships, many of them continuing in the bedroom next to her. Jane did not like any of the men her mother lived with, and much preferred the times when she had her mother to herself.

Friendships have always been a problem for Jane. During her life she has had a number of 'best friends', but, one way or the other, she feels they have all let her down. She has usually been one of a small group of girls on the estate, all of whom have had difficulties at home. From about the age of eleven, they have been part of a larger mixed group of children and then teenagers, who have hung around on the streets and got themselves a bad reputation with the residents and with the police. Jane attends the same comprehensive school as Mary, but they have no friends in common and mix in entirely different groups. None of the teenagers

Jane mixes with find school a rewarding place to be, and their best times are those they spend together in pubs, bars, and on the street. They all smoke, drink quite heavily, and do drugs, although none of them is dependent on drugs.

When she was twelve, shortly after her mother's boyfriend had attempted to molest her, Jane was taken behind one of the blocks of flats by a boy of fifteen who pushed her against the wall, lifted her skirt, pulled her knickers down and penetrated her. She had quite liked this boy, which is why she had gone behind the block with him. At this point in time, Jane was not fully developed physically. She found her first sexual experience painful and confusing. She promised herself she would not get into the same situation again. However about 15 months later, now fully developed, she had sex a number of times with a boy she liked, because he wanted it badly and she thought he would not go out with her any more unless she complied. He was rough with her, quite uninterested in whether she found the experience enjoyable, and indeed it never occurred to her she would. She was doing it for his pleasure, and found the whole process disgusting. In contrast to Mary, Jane has never masturbated and has had no sexual fantasies. Since that time, Jane has had sex with about 10 different boys and young men. She became pregnant on one occasion, and had no hesitation in having a termination.

Now, at seventeen, Jane has come across Henry, a man of twenty she really likes. She met him in a club a month ago. He works in his father's electrical goods shop. He has a lot of spare cash and drinks a good deal. She is employed as a checkout assistant in a supermarket and thinks about him a lot while she is working. Henry has a reputation as a bit of a lad, and she's worried about this, but she finds him attractive and, for the first time, finds herself quite interested in a man sexually. He has already tried to have sex with her, but she would really like to wait for some months before she agrees. But she knows he will lose interest in her if she tries this. She has spoken in a break to another girl at the supermarket, who has told her if she wants to keep him, she'll have to sleep with him, and soon. His friends will start to humiliate him if they learn he is going out with a girl who won't sleep with him.

These two vignettes are by no means at the extreme of sexual behaviour in the teens. There are many girls whose behaviour is much less advanced than that of Mary and others whose early sexual experience is even more unpleasant and unsatisfying than that of Jane.

Mary's development is fortunately much more typical of the way romantic relationships develop during the teen years in the western world. Most commonly there is a stage around 12–14 years when most sexual life is in fantasy. Masturbation frequently begins if it has not already occurred. Fantasies may involve celebrities and/or people, usually older people, drawn to the boy or girl. Short-lived romantic relationships lasting a few weeks and with little attempt at exclusiveness, often involving some physical contact, holding hands, then kissing and fondling, usually occur between 14 and 16 years. From 17–21 years romantic relationships are much more exclusive and, in the world of western adolescence, are likely to involve full sexual intercourse. Even by 21 years though, such relationships are unlikely to be permanent; they mainly last between one and three years.

But many young people have experiences much more like that of Jane. In many western countries about 1 in 4 young people has full sexual intercourse before the age of 16 years. Many who have sex at this age have less negative experiences than Jane but for some the experience is even more unpleasant.

6.3 **Variation is the pace of physical changes**

There is very wide variation in physical sexual development. This usually begins well before the teens. In both boys and girls, the first changes in sex hormone levels begin between five and nine years. In girls, there is a further significant increase in production of estrogens round about 9 or 10 years. The increase continues to about 13–14 years, by which time production has reached adult levels. So sex hormone secretion is at adult levels by the beginning of the teens; it doesn't continue to increase during this phase of life.

The range of ages at which bodily changes occur is vast. In girls, as a result of the increase in hormone secretion, changes in the shape of the breasts begin at any time between 8 and 13 years with the appearance of the 'breast bud'. Breast development is usually completed at any time between 13 and 18 years (average 15 years). The first menstrual period (menarche) can occur at any time between 10 and 17 years (average about 12 and a half years).

In boys, testosterone levels begin to rise at around 10 years and then rise sharply to reach adult levels at any time between 12 and 17 years, so it is not surprising that around the age of nine years, only about one in ten boys masturbate, but by thirteen years, this is true for eight out of ten. The scrotum and testes begin to enlarge and the scrotum darkens between 11 and 16 years. The adolescent spurt in height is usually completed by 16 years, though growth often continues until as late as 18 years. By the age of 15–16 years, most boys are physically mature and adult-like from the point of view of sexual development. Adult levels of sex hormones are reached during the teens but the idea that the levels are unusually high at this time is false.

There is no reason to think that the young are tormented by volcanic eruptions of hormonal lava that only subside in adult life. Both in boys and girls, the production of sex hormones is more uneven than it is in adult life and it often takes some months for menstruation to become regular, but levels of sex hormones are, in general, no higher in the teens than they are in later adult life. For young people in their mid and late teen years, the experience of adult levels of sex hormones with the resulting rise in intensity of sexual desire, is always new, sometimes confusing, sometimes purely pleasurable, and mostly a very mixed experience, but the hormone levels are no different from those found in young adults.

6.4 **Variations in sexual development**

So the teen years are by no means as special in sexual development as most people believe. Wide variation between individuals happens with all types of bodily change. Some men lose their hair and become bald in their twenties while others keep a thick thatch well into their old age. Some women experience the menopause in their thirties, while others are still seeing their periods in their fifties. These are much bigger variations than those that occur with the onset of puberty. Age variations matter more in the teens because teenagers are so strongly separated into groups by age. In school, where they spend so much of their lives, they are very strictly age-segregated. So comparisons, with others of the same age, at times gratifying, at times very painful, are inevitable.

The differences between adolescents during puberty are most noticeable round about the age of 12 years. At that age a girl may be fully developed physically. She will have started her periods a year or so earlier and it will now be regular in frequency. She will have nearly reached her adult height and her weight will have become redistributed so that she will have a rounded posterior with large breasts and a deep cleavage. Another girl in her class may only just be showing the first signs of puberty with breast budding that is not yet visible through her clothes. This girl may have to wait another two or three years for her periods to start and, though she will be taller, her body will still have the same shape it had when she was five years younger. She will not have started her adolescent growth spurt and may be a full 6 inches shorter than her early maturing classmate.

With boys, because they mature on average a year or two later, the age when differences between them is most marked is around 13 or 14 years. At that age some will be shaving once a day, have had their first ejaculation a couple of years previously, and be masturbating regularly. Others will look much as they did a few years back, just like little boys. Their growth spurt will not have occurred and the height difference between early and late maturers may be as much as 9 or 10 inches.

6.5 **Variations in the age of sexual maturity**

One of the myths about sex and the teens is that there was a large drop in the age when puberty began in the last half of the twentieth century. In fact, the age of puberty did indeed drop very rapidly in Western Europe much earlier during the nineteenth and first half of the twentieth century. In the mid-nineteenth century, the average age of menarche (the first menstrual period) in England was around 15 years and by the mid-twentieth century it was more like 12 and a half years. Similar changes occurred in the United States, Finland, Norway, and Italy. Why did this happen? The reason for this dramatic change, a drop of about a year for every half century, cannot be genetic. The population transmitted the same genes down the generations. There is much more likely to be a dietary explanation. Over that time period, children were much better nourished than they were in early Victorian times. That caused them not only to be taller, but also to mature earlier sexually. However this drop in the age of puberty stopped occurring about 50 years ago, probably because, by that time, most of the population was receiving an optimum diet. Although it is widely believed that children enter puberty earlier today than they did 30 or 40 years ago, evidence for this belief is, as Russell Viner has shown, very weak, and it seems likely there has only been a small change and, more probably no change at all.

Very different explanations have been found for the marked differences between children in the ages when they enter puberty? As with most variation in biology, the main reason here does lie in our genes. Identical twins of the same sex who share the same genes go through puberty within a month or two of each other. Non-identical twins who have shared the same environment but only share half their genes vary much more, often by a year or two. There is a strong relationship between the age a mother started her periods, and the age her daughter begins. Late maturing mothers have late maturing daughters. This could, of course, be because mothers and daughters have been brought up in similar social conditions, but the twin evidence is very compelling. Diet is also of significance. Well-nourished children start puberty before those who are deprived and disadvantaged. The social circumstances in which a child is brought up do also play at least a minor part. It used to be thought that children whose parents have divorced or separated went through puberty earlier, but this does not seem to be the case. What does seem to hold up in a number of different studies is that girls tend to mature a little earlier if their father has been absent from home during their earlier childhood. Why this should be is not at all clear, and there have been no convincing explanations.

6.6 **Variations in sexual orientation**

Only about 3% of adult men and about 1–2% of women are exclusively homosexual in adult life. Teenage boys are more likely to show such behaviour, especially if they go to single-sex secondary or boarding schools. So there must be a number of boys, perhaps about one in ten, who have homosexual relationships in adolescence, but stop during or immediately after their teens. The homophobia (a cause of so much unhappiness in gay teens), found in schools and discussed later in this chapter, not only prevents such boys 'coming out' in adolescence, but also encourages boys with some degree of in-built homosexuality to repress their sexual preference, often until much later in adult life when they may have married and had children.

6.7 **Understanding teenage sex**

Understanding the sexual behaviour of Jane and Mary involves knowing something about them as individuals, but even more about the values and attitudes of the social groups in which they live. In some groups nearly all girls have lost their virginity by the age of 17 years, while in others virtually all girls of this age remain sexually inexperienced. As we see in Chapter 2, in traditional societies there is a great range of attitudes to sexual behaviour in the teens, some being highly permissive, and others fanatically controlling. Orthodox Muslim, Hindu, and Jewish parents, and born-again Christians regard the preservation of the sexual purity of their daughters before marriage as their main parental responsibility. Indeed, paradoxically, girls brought up in an orthodox religious environment are much like Jane in the degree of choice they have in sexual matters. But whereas Jane feels she has no choice but to sleep with the boys and young men she meets, girls reared in religiously orthodox families have no choice but to retain their virginity. Their contacts with boys, if they have any, are strictly regulated so as to prevent any possibility of sexual activity.

When, one way or the other, standards of sexual behaviour are rigidly prescribed, the personalities and special situations of individual teenagers play little part in whether or not they are sexually active. But most adolescents in western society do not live in such societies. For teenagers like Mary and Charles, individual personality, personal appearance, and often unpredictable social events are of great importance. Mary is a shy adolescent, but not so shy that she is incapable of making a new relationship with Charles. If she had been just that much more socially inhibited, this relationship might well not have developed in the first place, and sexual activity would have been out of the question. There are many girls a good deal more inhibited than Mary for whom this would be the case. Or Mary might not have been conventionally good looking. She might have been unfashionably plump or have some physical impairment. Again this could have acted as a deterrent to the making of a sexual relationship. An extravert personality or unusual physical attractiveness would act in the opposite direction. And, where rules of teenage sexual behaviour are flexible, the chemistry of relationships will sometimes play an important part. A couple of 15-year-olds may have sex much earlier than they otherwise would, just because they happen to meet at a party and fall passionately in love with each other.

In most westernized countries the average age when boys and girls first start to kiss and get involved in sexual activity falling short of intercourse is around 13 years. By 14 or 15 years, many will have moved on to mutual masturbation, with some form of oral sex occurring to an increasing degree. Masturbation is virtually universal by mid-puberty in boys and occurs frequently, though by no means universally in girls. These pleasurable forms of behaviour are not harmful, though many parents disapprove of some of them. In particular, beliefs once widely held by doctors as well as the lay public that masturbation can produce blindness or madness have, of course, no basis in fact, though guilt about masturbation is still not uncommon and is fostered by some religious groups.

6.8 Is the age of first intercourse so much younger now?

It seems well established by the work of Kaye Wellings and her colleagues that, over the 50 years from the end of the Second World War in 1945, there was a dramatic change in the age at which full sexual activity took place in Britain. Among women reaching their teenage years between 1944 and 1948, the average age at first full intercourse was 21 years. For those reaching the age of 13 years between 1954 and 1958 it was 19 years, and it declined to 17 years for those reaching their teens between 1979 and 1988. The same story, though less dramatic, holds for boys. For boys reaching 13 years between 1944 and 1948, the average age at first intercourse was 19 years with a drop to 17 years for those reaching teen age between 1979 and 1988. During this time, the average age when girls had their first period dropped just about a month from 13 years 5 months to 13 years 4 months. It is clear that earlier physical maturation cannot go anywhere near explaining the drop in the age when girls had their first full sexual experience.

Although the last 50 years has seen a decline in the age of all forms of sexual behaviour in the western world, this is not a universal trend. There are large differences between social groups in the age of girls when virginity is lost. While there has been a decline in average age of first intercourse throughout the whole of the western world, this drop is either hardly noticeable or has not occurred at all in orthodox Jewish and Muslim groups, in southern Italy and Greece, or in the Baptist belt in the southern United States. It is increasingly difficult to identify places in the western world where virginity before marriage is still prized, but they certainly still exist, and they exist in places where puberty takes place at the same time as elsewhere.

Martin Richards has pointed out that the age of puberty and the hormonal changes that occur at the time of puberty, are only some and sometimes not the most important factors deciding when and to what degree, sexual behaviour occurs in the teenage population. Sexual intercourse may occur as normal, expected behaviour before puberty begins. When a team led by J. Richard Udry investigated sexual behaviour and its relation to puberty in American high school children, they decided to study young people aged over 13 and a half years. But as far as some groups of American teenagers were concerned, it turned out they had missed the boat. Most in these groups had already had sexual intercourse by the time the study began, in many cases *before* they had reached puberty.

In that case why has there been such a remarkable reduction in the age of intercourse in many sections of western society over the last 50 years? Virginity at marriage is much less prized than it was, but this begs the question why it now matters less to a young man and his family that his bride should not be a virgin. More mixed sex schools mean there are more opportunities for boys and girls to meet informally. Increased space in homes, with most adolescents now having a room of their own, means there is more privacy available to couples. With more families in which both parents work, — those in their teens are more often at home alone, left to their own devices. But boys and girls did meet before without too much difficulty and ways could always be found for privacy if that was what a couple wanted. The ready availability of contraception has doubtless made a real difference to the risk of pregnancy, itself a deterrent to sex before marriage. Although many teenagers do not use contraception when they have sex, this must be a significant factor. It is unlikely to be the sole cause because the age of intercourse was declining before safe contraception in the form of a pill was available, so there must be other reasons.

Probably all the factors mentioned have played some part, and there are others. Where adults lead the way, adolescents follow. It is now much more widely acknowledged than it used to be that women enjoy sexual pleasure as much as men. There was a widespread belief, lasting well after Victorian times that nice girls did not enjoy sex at least until they had been in love for months if not years, and were safely married. The media, films, television, and women's magazines have put paid to that idea and probably intimate discussion between women friends meant it never had much private credence anyway.

All the same, before the 1950s, many women did not regard it as their right to enjoy sexual pleasure. The feminist movement, with significant success, endeavoured to establish women's rights in all areas of life, including that of sexual freedom and the enjoyment of sex. Sex before marriage between adults has become not just more explicitly acceptable, but almost universally expected. In a British survey published in 1994, virtually all men and women aged 16–24 had had their first sexual experience before marriage. In those aged 45–59 over a third of women and one in seven men had their first such experience in marriage. Finally, though sexual relationships outside marriage have always occurred, increasing affluence, greater mobility, and many more opportunities for men and women to meet in the work place, have made it a great deal easier for them to develop.

6.9 Greater freedom – more risk

Although the focus of this book is on the teen years, the fact is that the more permissive relationships between the sexes that came about during the second half of the twentieth century, affected those in their twenties and thirties just as much, if not more, as it did those in their teens.

Changes in the sexual lives and, perhaps as importantly, changes in the non-sexual mixed-sex relationships of adolescents brought many benefits with them. Relationships between teenagers are richer, more open, and in many senses more rewarding. There is less sexual repression. Adolescents are better informed about sexual matters than they used to be. But alongside these benefits, a number of problems have increased considerably. These have arisen at least partly because the more permissive attitude to teenage sex has not been accompanied by information empowering young people to enjoy their greater sexual freedom safely. What are the dangers and how, as far as possible, can they be avoided?

6.9.1 Pregnancy: planned, half-planned, and unplanned

In the UK and much of the westernized world most young people have full sexual intercourse during their mid and late teenage years, when they are at their most fertile, and most have unprotected sex on some occasions, so it is surprising that unwanted pregnancy is still relatively uncommon. In England and Wales, only about one in thirty-five young women aged 15–19 years have a baby each year, and about one in fifty have an abortion. The rates are much lower in younger teenagers. Only about 1 in 250 13- to 15-year-olds have an abortion and about the same number have a baby each year. Of course, these numbers are too high, and they are higher in the UK than in most other western European country, though not as high as in the USA. An early pregnancy is not always unwanted, but it usually is. Having a baby in the mid and even the late teens results in missed education and therefore missed career opportunities.

For some girls who get pregnant, education is far from top of their priorities in life. More than anything else, perhaps because they have missed out in their early lives, they want to be loved and to have someone to love themselves. But the fact is that missing out on educational opportunities in adolescence reduces their choices in life, and many do regret this later on.

Sometimes, from the media, one would get the impression that half the teenage girl population is pregnant at any one time. In December 1999, a 17-year-old girl gave birth to twins fathered by a 13-year-old boy. The acres of column space dedicated to this incredibly unusual event gave the impression that this was a common occurrence. Such events can however be instructive. For example, it turned out that both sets of parents thought that a boy could not father a child until his sixteenth birthday, and there are messages here to do with the need for sex education. But the impression given that all over England, girls were having sex with boys in their early teens was totally misleading. In fact, the rate of abortion is higher in young adults, those in the 20–24 age group, than it is in older adolescents. So unprotected sex leading to unwanted pregnancy is actually commoner in young adults than it is in adolescents.

6.9.2 **Sexually transmitted diseases**

Most teenagers, even those who have frequent sexual intercourse, do not suffer from sexually transmitted diseases. But a substantial minority do. For example, in England and Wales, about 6 in every 1000 15–19-year-old girls attend a clinic with a new infection of chlamydia, the most common sexually transmitted infection, every year. It is thought that only about one in ten young women with this infection attends a clinic so the actual rate is more like six in every hundred. Chlamydia, although curable and perhaps one of the less serious of sexually transmitted infections, can cause serious disease, especially in women. Infertility and chronic abdominal pain are among the complications. Like gonorrhoea and herpes it is about as common in adolescents as it is in young adults. HIV infection appears to be more common in young adulthood than in adolescence but this is because of the greater delay between infection and diagnosis with this condition.

Now as virtually all teenagers know, condoms can greatly reduce the rate of both unwanted pregnancy and sexually transmitted infections. A great deal is known as to why condoms are so unreliably used. Paradoxically, they are less likely to be used when they are most needed; when young people are having sex with people they know rather little and have only recently met. They are more likely to be used when the partners have known each other for at least a few weeks. Most of those who write about the subject stress the risk-taking attitudes of adolescents and their feelings of invulnerability. But taking risks, which, as seen in the last chapter, is mainly related to the inexperience of teenagers and not an essential part of their nature, is much more difficult to avoid if there is a lack of opportunity to plan for having sex, if condoms are difficult to obtain, and if, above all, young people do not have the skills to negotiate with each other in a way that makes the use of a condom less embarrassing and more acceptable. Added to this is the lack of knowledge teenagers have about the availability of birth control services in their areas. In a study in Exeter, over half the 15-year-olds questioned either didn't know there was such a service or thought there wasn't one. With skills and knowledge, teenagers have the power to safeguard themselves against unwanted pregnancies and infection. Without them they are at considerable risk.

6.9.3 Sex with violence

Though the situation has changed considerably over the years, it is still the case that most girls in heterosexual relationships expect the boy to take the lead in progressing sexual activity. There comes a point when the girl does not wish to go further. She has often made up her mind before the action starts how far she wants to go. The boy then has three choices. He can accept the girl's decision, or he can bring what he regards to be gentle pressure to bear to proceed, desisting if he meets resistance, or he can use physical force to advance the action. Most people, including most adolescents would regard the use of gentle pressure as acceptable and the use of violence as definitely not. But situations are not so simple. Problems arise when what a boy regards as gentle pressure is seen by the girl as a threat of further violence if she does not comply.

Even in the minds of many adults, the distinction between rape and seduction is blurred and confused. The pronouncements of judges in cases of rape and attempted rape are often profoundly offensive to feminists and not only to feminists but to most women and at least some men. Some judges appear to believe that a woman who dresses attractively and goes to a man's flat is inviting intercourse and a man cannot be blamed if he uses force to achieve it, even if she makes it abundantly clear she does not want it. This view is shared by many men. So it is not surprising that teenagers are similarly confused. An Australian study found that one in three 14-year-old boys believed it was reasonable to rape a girl if she 'led him on'. In another study, two Australian researchers, Susan Moore and Deborah Rosenthal, surveying 16-year-old boys, found clear evidence of 'exploitative views about sexual relationships as well as aggression towards girls who were not sexually accommodating'. They pointed to 'a continuum in the boys' methods of achieving their sexual goals—methods which ranged from seemingly harmless persistence and titillation through to the clearly unacceptable techniques of derogation and force'. Asked whether he would try to persuade a girl to have sex if she didn't want to but he did, one typical response was, 'Yes, I would try. I would touch her and stare at her', but another, nearer the middle of the continuum said, 'I would try to persuade her, maybe with a bit of force. I wouldn't rape the girl, but kiss her and so on, touch her vagina, her bosoms, try to stimulate her, and if she didn't want to, I would just talk to her and see what is wrong'. Another 16-year-old just said, 'Sure, mate, shove it in' and yet another 'Yes, mate. Root the fucking bitch in the fucking arse'. Over two-thirds of the teenage boys interviewed said they would try to convince a reluctant female partner to have sex with them. Even allowing for some macho exaggeration, these statements suggest a remarkable level of expectation of violence in sexual relationships among young males.

Discussion of sexual abuse of young teenagers is usually limited to situations where much older men, often fathers or stepfathers, are involved. Of course, this does happen, and much more than it should. But in a much more common scenario older teenage boys force slightly younger girls to have sex with them. This is much more problematic from both a moral and a legal point of view, and may be no less traumatic as far as girls are concerned. A 17-year-old boy who forces a 15-year-old physically mature girl to have sex with him against her will, is unlikely to land up in court, or to meet with the disapproval of his friends or even of his parents. Yet the distress to the girl may be considerable. But we must not forget that it is the tolerant adult attitudes towards men who forcibly pressure women to have sex with them that provide most of the explanation for the attitudes and sometimes the confusion of teenagers.

6.9.4 **The trivialization of sex**

In previous generations, sexual intercourse, especially the first full sexual experience, was almost universally regarded as a 'big deal'. This view is now relatively uncommon. Among some groups of young people, if a couple are attracted to each other, sex is likely to occur at the first or second meeting. 'Shagging' has much the same level of significance as sharing a meal or going to a cinema together. Compared to its former status as an event of major, if not momentous significance, it has become trivialized. Among both adults and teenagers, sexual activity between consenting partners is widely regarded as a morally acceptable activity if it takes place in a relationship to which neither partner feels even a short-term commitment. Of course, many do not hold this view, and even among those who do, most would agree that it is more desirable, more pleasurable and, in a sense, more moral, for sex to take place between partners who care for each other and see themselves in a long-term relationship. But teenagers generally do not expect themselves to be in such long-term relationships. So their alternatives are between no sex, sex falling short of intercourse, and full but trivialized sexual activity. The last option was well put by Karl, the teenager in the American film 'Election'. At a crisis in his life, he prays and thanks God for the good parts of his life. One good part, he says, is that most people think he has a pretty big penis. Another is that he and his girlfriend go back to his house three or four times a week 'for a burger and a fuck'; for Karl there is no irony in this equation.

Such trivialization of sex, though now common, may lead to experiences that are regretted. A study by Danny Wight of 14-year-old Scottish girls who had had a full sexual experience, revealed that about half of those they interviewed either thought their first experience of sexual intercourse was too early or that it should never have taken place at all. Regret was especially likely to be expressed if the sex had occurred as a result of pressure or of being pressured. It is, of course, equally interesting that about half these 14-year-olds thought their first experience of intercourse had occurred 'at about the right time'.

6.9.5 Family arguments

When boys and girls in their early and mid-teens develop intense sexual relationships, their parents often disapprove. They may disapprove of their child having such a relationship at all, or, just as commonly, they disapprove of their child's choice of partner. Violent arguments sometimes follow, with the whole family affected by anger, frustration, and depression. This is the scenario often identified when a teenager is brought into an Accident and Emergency Department having attempted suicide. In many cases, the family has been torn apart by arguments for years, and the sexual relationship is just a new focus for disharmony. But the introduction of a sexual element into the situation frequently brings with it a new intensity to the family discord. It all seems to matter much more. When sexual relationships start for the first time later in adolescence this fits more readily into the parents' expectations for, by this time, the young person has already established an acceptable level of independence in other areas of life.

If early sex brings with it sexual violence, abortion and unwanted pregnancies, sexually transmitted diseases, and an increase in the intensity of family arguments, it sounds like an event youngsters under sixteen could well do without! But this is not a view taken by many in their early teens, especially teenage boys. Doubtless many parents do succeed in warning their children off early sex, but it is clear many don't, and it is not hard to see why. When moral disapproval has been removed from sex outside marriage, when the opportunities for young people to meet in unsupervised situations have increased so much, when messages from the media are all in the direction of encouragement of sexual activity, and when young people live in such a highly sexualized climate, it is surprising sexual behaviour in the early teens is not more widespread than it is.

A comparison carried out by Dr Roger Ingham, of the University of Southampton, between young people in Holland and the UK provides helpful information. In Holland the teenage birth rate has consistently been one of the lowest in Europe, while that in the UK has been one of the highest. In Holland sex education usually begins in primary school. Abortion is free and easily accessible. There is open discussion of sexual issues in young people on television and radio. Dutch teenagers only, on average, have sexual intercourse a little later than British, but they are much more likely to have known their partner for longer, to have discussed the issue of contraception before intercourse, and to have used a condom on this occasion. Dutch young people are more likely to have their first full sexual experience with someone with whom they fell in love and to whom they feel emotionally committed. Only about 1 in 7 UK males felt in love or emotionally committed to the person they first had intercourse with, compared with nearly half the Dutch males. Physical attraction and peer pressure were much more important factors for UK than for Dutch couples. The Dutch are more likely to have had the opportunity for mixed sex relationships early on and to confide in young people of the opposite sex as much as their own sex. Further, Dutch teenagers are more likely to have talked about sex with one or both parents before they have sex. Their parents are more likely to have shown open physical affection and warmth to each other. It is impossible to explain fully the differences between the pregnancy rates of Dutch and British teenagers from this information. But it does seem likely that the more open attitudes to sexual matters and the early sex education play some part. Similarly the later age of first sexual intercourse in French teenagers has been attributed to better communication about sex between family members.

In contrast, preaching the evils of early sex seems to make very little difference. The more one gives adolescents the power to make decisions about their own sexual behaviour, the less dangerous and the more sensible those decisions are likely to be.

6.10 Sex: protection, preparation, and then empowerment

There are two major ways in which our society is confused in the messages it provides to children and young people as far as their sexual behaviour is concerned. Our first major inconsistency lies in the fact that the law states that it is an offence for a young man to have sex, even if she is a willing partner, with a girl under the age of 16 years. Yet survey evidence suggests that around one-third of 14- and 15-year-olds have had intercourse. Now most, if not all, adults would think that it would be better if 14- and 15-year-old girls did not have sex. Yet, from about the age of seven or eight years, many girls in our society are encouraged to dress both seductively and provocatively. We allow them to wear T-shirts with suggestive messages like 'So Many Boys, So Little Time'. They wear lipstick and nail varnish. Discos are arranged for them at which, often unsupervised, they have access to alcohol and plenty of opportunity to experiment sexually with others of the same age. When they go to parties, parents are often complicit in encouraging them to wear sexually provocative clothes. This 'tweeny' phase of development from about 9-13 years has been commercially created and exploited by those in the fashion business, but parents, pressured by their young, go along and are sometimes encouraging.

Our second major inconsistency is that we permit a situation in which young people reach an age when we accept many of them are going to have sex without anything like adequate preparation for the emotionally powerful experiences they will probably find both enjoyable and distressing. Further, although we know that sexual activity can be dangerous, though much more is being done than was the case even a decade ago, we still do far too little to make sure they are adequately equipped to deal with such hazards.

Both these inconsistencies need addressing. And they can only be properly addressed if adult society collectively makes up its mind about two issues. As we have seen, a substantial minority of 14–15-year-olds are having sex. Much can be done to discourage those as young as this from sexual activity, but it is not reasonable to think the adult world can stop it. Nor is it sensible to have a law that is so frequently broken with impunity. On the other hand, is it in any way acceptable for girls and boys under the age of 14 years to have full sexual experience? If not, what can we do about it? Further, if it is inevitable, though undesirable at least until later in the teens, for girls and boys from the age of 14 upwards to have full sexual experience, how can we try to ensure both that those young people who have reached the age of 14 years are as well prepared as possible for the experience, and that such preparation does not make it more likely that others will engage in what we agree is an undesirable behaviour?

What follows are suggestions as to what we might do if we really do believe first, that it is unacceptable for children under the age of 14 years to have sex and second, that young people aged 14 years and over should be adequately prepared for the experience, even though many of us believe it is desirable for full sexual intercourse to be delayed at least until the last half of the teen years.

6.11 **Preparing the under 14s for but protecting them from full sexual relationships**

Early relationships. The first steps in preparation for sexual relationships are taken at home within the family in the very early years of life. Children do not reach their teen years in a naïve and unformed state, but bring a great deal of experience as well as skill with them into their teenage years. Most importantly, as far as relationships and sex are concerned, they bring experiences of care and friendship. With one or both parents, unless they have been unlucky, they will have developed a mutually affectionate relationship. Within this relationship, they will have learned how to be cared for and how to care. Their relationship with their parents will have given them a sense of boundaries, of the fact that some behaviour is permitted and some not. As I discussed in Chapter 3, they will have come to understand both from arguing with their parents and from observing what happens when their parents disagree with each other, that, when conflicts arise, they can be settled by negotiation. There will be many other aspects of their relationships with their parents, such as the way they manage to cope with separation from them, and how they deal with feelings of envy and jealousy about them. These experiences will have equipped them with rich knowledge and skill, now called 'emotional intelligence', even before they arrive at adolescence. Such children will stand a good chance of being able to deal by negotiation with the new challenges posed by their first serious encounters with the opposite sex.

But, as again I have indicated in Chapter 3, they may not have been so lucky. At the other extreme, children entering adolescence may have had parents who, for one reason or another, have not been able to provide anything like adequate care. They may have experienced frequent separations from their own parents with spells in children's homes or foster care. As an everyday event, they may have seen their parents drunk or drugged and settling conflicts by beating each other up. They may themselves have been beaten as a matter of course when they have not done what their parents wanted and know no other way of resolving differences.

When, for one reason or another, children have not been cared for well, this rapidly shows in their sexual behaviour once they reach adolescence. There is a striking illustration of this in the sexual fate of children who have been taken into the long-term care of social services departments because their parents have been unable to look after them. One in four of the girls in this situation are mothers by the age of eighteen, compared with less than one in thirty in children brought up in family care. One study showed that two-thirds of male prostitutes have been brought up in children's homes.

Between the extremes of excellent care and gross neglect, children will have had a range of more or less good caring experiences, all of which will have had an influence on how well equipped they are to deal with new relationships, especially sexual relationships, on entering their teenage years.

Depending largely on the quality of care they have received in the early years of their lives, but also on their personalities and on the sort of friends they happen to make at primary school and in their neighbourhoods, children develop skills in making and keeping friendships, and in negotiating successfully the conflicts that inevitably arise in relationships. Children who reach their teenage years without the capacity for sustained relationships will be ill-equipped to deal with the new lives they are expected to lead. This means that anything that is done to improve the social skills and knowledge of children in their pre-teens, with both the same and the opposite sex, will help them cope better with the sexually charged encounters they are quite likely to experience once they reach their early and mid-teen years. They will feel more in charge, and indeed they will be.

Avoidance of premature sexualization. When 7–8-year-old girls are encouraged to use lipstick, put on brightly coloured nail varnish, and wear T-shirts with sexually suggestive messages, the assumption must surely be that it is perfectly acceptable for girls of this age to have regular boyfriends to whom they are sexually attractive and with whom they can have sexual fun. It would surely be preferable for the adult world to take a strong line and discourage such premature sexualization. There is, as every adult knows, a fine line between, on the one hand dressing attractively and, on the other, dressing provocatively and seductively, just as there is between behaving in an attractive and charming manner and behaving in a manner specifically designed to 'pull'. The fact that drawing this distinction in the way one looks and behaves is a social skill means that children need to acquire it.

Monitoring and supervision by parents. One of the best indicators whether children engage in premature sexual activity, as well as virtually any other undesirable activity, is the level of monitoring and supervision their parents exercise. Now this makes it sound as though parents have to keep their eyes on their children the whole time. Everyone knows that is just not possible. Further, as we see in Chapter 3, a highly restrictive or authoritarian approach to bringing up children merely succeeds in making them more likely to break important rules. Why then does monitoring turn out to be so important? Probably the reason is that the essential part of 'monitoring' is not constant surveillance, but in parents taking a real interest in what their children are doing, being able to discuss where they are going and how they are going to behave, and only very occasionally exercising a veto.

Curiosity about sex leads nearly all children into sexual experimentation long before puberty begins. The excitement that comes with the prohibited inspection and sometimes cautious touching of the genitalia of other children, perhaps in games of doctors and nurses, makes experimentation irresistible. Most parents sensibly feel that if they come across such activity it is better to take an indulgent but mildly discouraging attitude, thus preventing it going further but also avoiding the implication that sexual activity is wicked. Once children reach the ages of 12 or 13 years, they may well be involved in affectionate kissing, to which most parents take a similar view. However, if they discover their children engaged in more serious sexual activity, especially but not only if it is accompanied by coercion, a permissive attitude borders on neglect and lack of adequate supervision.

Encouragement to make friends with other children of both sexes. Children will find it easier to make intimate, caring relationships once they reach their mid-teens if they have made friends with others of both sexes in their earlier lives. Boys and girls are indeed different, and they are made more different by their upbringing, but they do not come from species alien to each other. If the first contacts boys and girls make with each other are in the context of the sexual chase, it surely makes it more difficult for them to enjoy each other's company. Life is made more difficult than it need be by attendance at single-sex schools at primary level. Both parents and teachers can encourage, though they will not be able to force mixed-sex friendships in the pre-teen years.

6.12 Home and school: telling children about sex in the primary years

From the time that children enter infant school, both protection against premature sexual activity and preparation for the time when it can safely be expected to begin becomes the responsibility of both parents and teachers. In primary school, children are now expected to be taught first about the names of the main parts of the body, rules for keeping safe, and people who can help them if they begin to feel unsafe, as well as to listen to, play with, and cooperate with others. Later, while still at primary school age, they need to be taught about the changes in emotions that puberty brings and how to manage these emotions, about the risks in different situations, and what kind of contact is acceptable and what unacceptable, as well as about different types of relationships.

One useful way for parents to think about how they can help to make sexual matters easier for their children is for them to work out early on, long before their children reach their teens, what their attitudes are to this part of life. Do they believe that girls should keep their virginity for as long as possible, whereas boys should lose theirs as rapidly as possible? Do they think that ado-lescence is a time for sexual experimentation and sleeping around as much as possible before stable relationships are entered upon, or that it is preferable for sex only to occur once such a relationship has been established? It is better to have thought about these matters early rather than to go into panic mode when children first start to show serious interest in sexual activity. If parents differ, as they well may, it is as well to try to work out a common front before puberty arrives rather than when it has started. This is not to say that their chil-dren will necessarily share parents' attitudes. Young people in their early teens develop their own ideas from a variety of sources, including especially their friends and what they see slightly older people doing. But they also appreciate it when they know what their parents' beliefs are. They may not want to be steered, but they do like to know what their parents think about these matters.

Most parents will not be concerned about sexual behaviour falling short of intercourse. But it is likely that they will want their children to have inter-course only when they are in a loving relationship. They will probably know from their own experience that this is sometimes difficult. Physical attraction often occurs without any sort of affectionate relationship and is difficult to resist. Parents may want to be honest about that. Although it may seem too obvious to mention, most parents will want their children to find sex pleasur-able, not painful or distressing which, as we have seen, for young people in their teens, it sometimes is. Parents may want their children to know that any-thing that happens between two people sexually is acceptable, providing they both want to do it and it's safe. Violence in sex and sex that risks health or unwanted pregnancy, they may wish their children to believe, is definitely not acceptable. They may also want their children to know however that sexual behaviour falling short of intercourse can be highly pleasurable and involves fewer health and emotional risks.

Many parents find it difficult to talk to their children about sexual matters. They are embarrassed themselves and their children often discourage them if they broach the subject. Offers to have 'a little chat' about sex are often met with a rushed 'It's all right. I don't need to, I know all about it'. And indeed some young people in their teens do indeed probably know more than their parents, though many don't and all would benefit from some communication on the subject. Parents are more likely to be successful if they first establish themselves, perhaps while watching television, as people who still find some members of the opposite sex attractive. Then when the action heats up in love scenes, they can make remarks conveying information about different forms of contraception. They might even say something like 'I hope she remembers to go to the chemist tomorrow morning for her morning after pill'. This may be met with 'I know what you're getting at and you can just shut it.' But the point may be worth making all the same! Such an interchange also makes it clear that parents are happy to talk about sexual matters if their children wish it.

As their children reach the teenage years, most parents are going to find it too difficult to talk to their own children about some of the practical aspects of lovemaking, for example how to put on a condom, for boys how to delay orgasm, and for girls how to achieve it. They should receive such information at school, and most now do. Such information is now also readily available from magazines for teenagers, mostly in a form at least as accurate as that their children will pick up from friends. Some information parents can provide, such as the address of the local family planning clinic if their children are unlikely to go to their GP for contraceptive advice. They can also assure their children that if they do go to the GP, they can be sure that the consultation will be confidential. They will only talk to the GP if they, their children, want them to. Young people are often concerned about the degree of confidentiality for which GPs can be relied on, and, sadly, their concerns are occasionally well founded.

6.13 **Home and school: discussing sex in the teen years**

So much for the pre-teen years, or at least for those below the age of 15 or 16 years. Once young people reach this age, they need to be sexually empowered, not so that they can be free to have multiple sexual relationships, though doubtless a minority will, but so that they can make good choices in their relationships and how to conduct them. To many parents, teachers, and members of the general public, the idea of encouraging the sexual empowerment of young people in their teens will seem ludicrous. Surely, they will say, adolescents are already sexually powerful enough. But this is to accept that the media messages of a raunchy, promiscuous teenage generation at their face value. Interviews with those in their teens, even those quite late in their teens, suggest that, for some, the reality is the very opposite of this picture. A minority remain sexually ignorant but many do not have the life skills to act on the knowledge they do possess. The rate of unplanned pregnancies and sexually transmitted infections is evidence of this, if any is needed. Although some will be ignorant of the physical side of sex, there is a good evidence most will be quite well informed about this side of things. A survey of 15-year-olds carried out in 1999 suggested that less than 10% felt they did not know enough about how their bodies developed. But one in four felt they had not received enough information about sexual feelings and emotions. When it came to practical aspects of sex, more than one in five thought they needed to know more about the use of a condom. Interestingly the subjects on which these 15-year-olds felt they had been kept most in the dark were lesbianism and homosexuality, and I shall discuss this issue later in the chapter.

But what these young teenagers are mainly lacking is the ability to negotiate with each other so that they each get what they really want. And what do they want? For girls it is most likely to be an intimate, confiding relationship, a feeling of being cared for, and the social status of having a boyfriend. For boys, it is all of these and, in addition, the release of sexual tension and, with that, some affirmation of their masculine status. Neither boys nor girls want to father or mother a baby, nor, even less, do they want to pick up a disease. Now anyone with sexual knowledge and some experience of negotiation in relationships knows that it is quite possible for all these aims to be achieved.

Here are some letters from teenagers in one issue of 'Bliss', a magazine mainly aimed at girls in their mid-teens. This magazine has four separate pages for readers' letters. They are devoted to love dilemmas, life troubles, sex questions, and body worries. These letters are taken from life troubles and sex questions. I expect some of them were made up by the editorial staff. But even if this is the case, presumably the staff at Bliss have a good idea of the issues teenagers worry about.

1. I feel trapped by my parents' rules. The more they refuse to let me date boys, wear make-up and stay out, the more I want to push the limits. Why do they treat me like a child? Miserable, 16, Birmingham.

2. I'm 16 and I think I might be gay. I'm not interested in boys and lately I've been attracted to girls and women. I'm afraid of what my mates might think if I tell them but I don't know what else to do. Confused, 16, Southampton.

3. My friends say masturbating can ruin your chances of having babies. Is this true? Concerned, 15, Cornwall.

4. My boyfriend has asked me to give him a 'wank', but I don't know how to. Can you explain what to do? Naïve, 17, Dundee.

5. I'm thinking of sleeping with my boyfriend and I'd like to talk to someone about contraception, but I can't see my GP as he's a close family friend. Will he tell on me? Cautious, 15, Manchester.

Such letters, together with information obtained from surveys carried out by the Brook Centres and the Trust for the Study of Adolescence suggest a high level of ignorance. We know that many girls in their mid-teens are a great deal better informed and have already embarked on a promiscuous sexual career. But even where promiscuity does occur, it is often accompanied by a good deal of distressing hurt and heartache. Many adolescents, like Jane in the account given above, feel, in their sexual lives, at the mercy of powers, both in themselves and in the world in which they live, over which they have little control. What is the cause of this sense of feeling of powerlessness, and how can it be overcome?

6.13.1 Sexual dilemmas of the teen years

When children move into their teenage years and become adolescents they face quite different amounts of 'sexual charge' at school and among their friends. Many will be living in a highly sexualized environment, partying every weekend, in which there is a strong expectation of early pleasurable sexual activity, while for some this is neither expected nor particularly desired. All the same, most 13- and 14-year-olds quite like the idea of having a special friend of the opposite sex, and it is surely natural that they should. For both boys and girls, a special friendship of this type brings status and a new, special source of pride and self-esteem. Girls hope especially to have an intimate, confiding type of relationship and someone else to care for. Boys, who will also gain status from having a special girlfriend, will be more interested in sharing activities. For both boys and girls the amount of investment in the relationship and its importance in their lives will depend on what else they have going for them. If school is going well and schoolwork is a source of self-esteem, or if, especially as far as boys are concerned, they are heavily involved in sport, having this new type of relationship will be an added bonus in life, but no more than that. But 13 and 14 years is often a time when young people become seriously alienated from school, and some have very little satisfaction from other aspects of their lives. For these, this new type of relationship may become desperately important.

This will be even more the case for children who feel deprived of affection at home. For boys in this group it is often important to their insecure status, not only that they have a girlfriend, but that they can 'score'. Girls who are deprived will find it difficult to say 'no' to penetrative sex if they think they are at risk of losing their boyfriend. He may not be the most caring individual, but he may be the only person who really 'wants' her. What is not possible is for a relationship that has all these desirable qualities to be lost without a great deal of distress. It is here that the social situation of adolescents puts them in a real quandary. They want a caring relationship, but, for a whole variety of reasons, their relationships are likely to be relatively short. The average length of boy–girl 'serious' friendships is around three to five months. Some are much shorter than this. Occasionally, teenage sweethearts get married in their late teens or early twenties and live to enjoy their diamond wedding anniversaries. But these are the rare exceptions. Much more commonly one of the pair is attracted to someone else. In a mixed school the opportunities for making other relationships is so great it would be surprising if break-up were any less frequent than it is. But the relationship may break up for other reasons. One of the families may move, for example, or one of the pair may lose interest in the friendship because they do not find it as rewarding as they did. So teenagers can either settle for relationships that are relatively unrewarding because they do not have any significant degree of commitment, or they can commit themselves in the knowledge that they are very likely to get badly hurt emotionally. They are poorly prepared and quite unable to cope with the mixture of emotions— the passion, love, pleasure, frustration, disappointment, anxiety, grief, envy, and jealousy—that may form part of a sexual relationship. Incidentally, it would be wrong to think of these dilemmas as 'teenage' problems. Young men and women in their twenties and thirties, and there are many of them, who are not in a stable relationship, though they may have been in one in the past, are in a very similar predicament. So are those in their forties and fifties who have divorced or lost a partner through death after a long-term relationship.

6.13.2 Helping teenagers take charge of their sexual lives: the role of teachers

There are many reasons why school needs to be the main source of information for young people in their teens. There is a frequent outcry over the fact that the number of births to teenage mothers is higher in the UK than it is in most other western European countries. This is indeed regrettable but we can do something about it. At the present time, we are failing to make knowledge and access to contraception available to young people as well as those in other countries. Only 50% of young people in Britain use contraceptives when they first have sex. In Denmark and Switzerland, the figure is nearer 80% and in the Netherlands, where sex education is much more explicit and interactive, it is nearer 85%.

The fact that unwanted sexual activity often occurs as a result of pressure and the implicit threat of violence is also relevant to the need for teachers to be engaged in sex education. Much more often than it should, sex in the teen years takes place when one partner, nearly always the boy or young man, gets his way by using more than gentle persuasion. Pressured sex can take many forms. At one extreme is emotional blackmail. As one girl described by Holland and colleagues put it, talking about an experience when she was fourteen and the man concerned was seventeen, '… I don't actually remember having any memory of saying to myself "this is what I want to do". I just remember doing it and thinking "it's not much of a big deal"… It just happened. I just accepted it'. A little further along the line is physical intimidation. To quote, '… I tried to push him off the bed. But every time I pushed him he pulled my hair. He said, 'if you don't let me, I'm going to pull your hair'. And finally there is rape.

Sexual violence is not an isolated form of violence. It occurs more easily in situations when violence is permitted or expected. This is seen most clearly in time of war when soldiers who have been expected to kill come across defence-less women. But it also happens in American schools when the level of violence is high. In general those who engage in physical violence in school against other students are also those most likely to rape. But sometimes it is not these boys or young men who rape, but the apparently timid or weak. These are students who have watched violence, wanted to participate, but been too frightened, and then, when they are not getting their way in a sexual encounter, model the behaviour they have witnessed on someone physically weaker than themselves.

One way of preventing sexual harassment and violence is therefore to pursue policies that reduce violence in schools more generally. Anti-bullying policies, described in Chapter 9, which are gradually being introduced, with more or less success into schools in Western Europe and North America, can therefore play a significant part in protecting young people, especially girls and young women, from rape and lesser forms of sexual intimidation.

Finally, there is the need to tackle the fact that, for many adolescents life is so lacking in other sources of self-esteem that trivialized sex, even unsafe sex, even pregnancy, and motherhood seem the only ways to achieve any form of pleasure out of life. Schools can and do play a major part in helping to empower and meet the needs of those teenagers who find learning so unrewarding.

6.13.3 Does sex education make sexual activity more likely?

Increasingly therefore teachers are taking responsibility for the sex education of those in their teen years. As we have seen, in the UK, though this is much less the case in Holland, many parents find it too difficult to talk to their teenage children or, just as frequently, their children find it too difficult to talk to them. During the 40 years between 1950 and 1990, the amount of sex education delivered in schools went up considerably. This was also the time, as we have seen, when the age of intercourse went down by three or four years. So was this the effect of more sex education, or were other factors, such as the availability of condoms and other forms of birth control, or the more explicit treatment of sex in the media or the increasing number of parental marriages breaking down more important?

Some light was thrown on this question by those who carried out the study mentioned earlier who found such a sharp drop in the age of first intercourse in British young people between 1950 and 1980. They found that, after taking into account other factors, those who received their main information about sex from school were actually likely to start sex later. School sex education delayed the age of intercourse. So it seems that changes in society were responsible for the drop in the age of first intercourse. Education about sex in schools probably prevented the drop being as great as it otherwise would have been.

Some confirmation of this finding was obtained from a study carried out in Exeter between 1991 and 1994. Over 1100 12–16-year-olds were given six lessons by a senior teacher assisted by a doctor. Physical aspects of sex and intercourse as well as skills in negotiation and assertiveness training were covered. In addition, the subjects had the opportunity of discussions about sex led by somewhat older teenagers. The knowledge of the teenagers and their likelihood of starting to have intercourse was then compared over the next three years both with young people in local schools and with others from a more distant locality that did not have this special intervention. The teenagers who had received systematic and authoritative sex education as well as discussion with older adolescents were distinctly more knowledgeable. Further, those in the control population were one and a half times more likely to have started intercourse than those who had had the intervention.

It is clear therefore that sex education focusing on relationships as well as the physical aspects of sex results in teenagers does not result in the young having sex earlier, and may even delay when first intercourse occurs. The lessons in Exeter were given by skilled health professionals. One could not guarantee the same outcome with less informed or less skilled teachers and there is evidence from Bristol that the quality of teaching makes a real difference. In the UK at the present time, sex education is supposed to occur within the science national curriculum. But science teachers are often poorly prepared to give lessons in the subject. It seems much more appropriate for sex education to occur in lessons specifically dedicated to personal, social and health education (PSHE). Although school inspectors are expected now to monitor the quality of PSHE lessons, the subject does not form part of the National Curriculum and thus has less status than it should. Further, following the 1993 Education Act, parents have the right to withdraw their children from any sex education that does not involve the biological aspects. Only about 1% of parents exercise this right, but it is likely that the fact that the right exists deters teachers from being as open about the non-biological aspects of sex as they would like to be.

6.13.4 Personal, social and health education (PSHE): the Cinderella subject

Teaching PSHE is not easy. As we shall see in Chapter 9, interactive education in secondary schools is, in general, more effective than straightforward lecturing. Many teachers are embarrassed or find it difficult to allow the expression of different views from students, some of which they profoundly disagree with. Yet unless the lessons are interactive, there is a good evidence, at least from the drugs field, that classes will risk being ineffective and a waste of time. Allowing free discussion of relationships is a sensitive task. Yet somehow or other teachers do need to impart the skills needed to make, maintain, and leave relationships without being cajoled, forced, or bullied into activities they really feel unhappy about. Some succeed in this, but training for teachers in the subject is almost non-existent, and, not surprisingly, many feel lacking in confidence in this area of their work.

6.13.5 Information about diversity of sexual orientation: homosexuality

In the current climate this is a very difficult issue for both parents and teachers. Parents may feel passionately that they do not want their children to turn out gay or lesbian. All other things being equal, most would agree that life is more problematic for gays and lesbians than it is for heterosexuals who can so readily be regarded as 'normal'. But bearing in mind there is now strong evidence that parents have very little control over the sexual orientation of our children, and that most will want to remain friends with their children whatever their sexual orientation, it is as well for parents to show tolerance of different forms of sexuality and to show they disapprove of any stigmatizing on this account.

Homosexuality poses even more difficult issues for teachers. Currently, the use of terms such as 'gay' and 'poofter' are among the most commonly used terms used by both primary and secondary age children as humiliating insults. Even children in infant school, who have a very limited understanding of homosexuality, use the terms in this way, to humiliate unpopular members of the class. Round about the ages of 13–15 years, about one in twenty boys will realize that they are only sexually attracted to others of the same sex. An additional uncertain number are attracted to both sexes, but gradually develop a heterosexual orientation. The homophobia that is widespread in schools means that these young people are forced to keep silent about their sexual feelings, while pretending to be the same as everyone else. There is ample anecdotal evidence about them finding this painful and distressing.

Until recently, the existence of Section 28 of the 1988 Local Government Act meant that local authorities could not promote homosexuality. Teachers have interpreted this as meaning they are not allowed to educate about homosexuality. Teaching about homosexuality is going to be difficult given the climate of homophobia in schools, but the repeal of this Section will make it a great deal easier to do so. If children are humiliated on account of their race or religion, teachers are strongly encouraged to take a strong line and, if all else fails, they are compelled by law to take action. While it might not be acceptable to pass similar legislation with respect to homosexuality, it is surely objectionable that cruelty relating to sexual orientation is so widely condoned, or at least ignored, in schools.

6.14 What the adult world could do to prepare, protect, and ultimately empower the young in their sexual lives

A useful first step would be for the adult world to stop putting out confusing messages about what it regards as appropriate sexual behaviour in children and those in their teens. It is clearly undesirable for girls under the age of 14 years to engage in sexual activity that might lead to intercourse.

On the other hand, once young people have reached about the age of 14 years, although it would clearly also be undesirable for the great majority of them to have intercourse not only because of the dangers to which I have already referred but because, in addition, they are poorly equipped to handle the emotions such activity arouses, some will be fully physically mature and will have started a caring and loving relationship with an older boy. If such a girl has intercourse, is it sensible to criminalize her boyfriend? Would it not be preferable instead to prepare her effectively? How then can the under 14s be protected against sexual activity and the over 14s empowered to choose whether to have sex and, if they do, as at least a small minority will, to protect them against the dangers?

So a second way in which the adult world can assist is to provide universal, high quality sex education in schools. At the moment, PSHE in schools is not an obligatory part of the National Curriculum. Clearly it should be. Although the Office for Standards in Education (Ofsted) has made it compulsory to monitor the PSHE components of the education of secondary schoolchildren, resources are too limited to provide it adequately. What is needed is a considerable increase in the number of trained PSHE teachers.

The adult world should also take seriously the fact that it would make the task of imparting information and skills to those in their teens easier if the age of consent was lowered from 16 to 14 years. It is not likely that legislation in this field would lead to any more or any less sexual behaviour. When 15-year-old girls refuse to have sexual intercourse with their boyfriends they do not do so because they are underage, but for a whole variety of other reasons, notably fear of the emotional consequences, fear of unwanted pregnancy, and fear of getting an unsavoury reputation.

Legislation to reduce the age of consent would make the task of talking about sex to secondary schoolchildren much less loaded with the possibility that the parent or teacher is actually encouraging a criminal act. Most young people think the age of consent is currently set too high. In a survey carried out in the year 2000, about 85% of girls aged 12–16 favoured a lower age limit. They are probably right. In Canada, Germany, Italy, and many other European countries with a lower teenage birth rate than the UK, the age of consent is 14 years, both for heterosexual and for homosexual behaviour. While the law is enforced incredibly rarely in this respect, it would also be sensible to remove from the realm of criminal activity, though of course not from the realm of what is regarded as quite unacceptable, sexual activity involving under 14-year-olds, providing there was mutual consent and there was no more than a three year gap between the two children involved. Such a sliding scale operates in Germany, Israel, and Switzerland without any problem, and it is difficult to see why it should not work in the UK. It would bring the law much closer to what happens in the real world, surely a desirable outcome. Sadly, at the time of writing in late 2003, a reverse legislative trend is occurring in England and Wales. The Sexual Offences Bill, largely drafted with the aim of protecting children against paedophiles, alas contains sections making 'sexual touching' a criminal offfence if one of the participants is under 16 years of age. It is difficult to see how a law that is so at variance with the behaviour of young people and that, in theory at least, criminalizes large numbers, probably most of them, can do other than create confusion in their minds and those of their parents.

Lowering the age of consent would also make it easier to provide the means of contraception to those currently under-age girls who are having unprotected intercourse but who do wish to obtain the means to protect themselves. Accessibility to confidential sexual health advice is difficult enough for 16–18-year-olds. Often young people do not know where to get such advice. The problems are much greater for girls who are currently underage. Chemists are not allowed to provide emergency contraception to them. Many general practitioners are reluctant to help and those who do are often unclear in the degree of confidentiality they practice, so that girls are uncertain whether their parents will be told about consultations they make. By acting in this way, the adult world seems to be acting less responsibly than the young who wish to protect themselves against unwanted pregnancy. That cannot be right.

6.15 Young people's views about sexual health services

Young people in their teens often wish to consult a doctor, a nurse, or a counsellor confidentially, especially about sexual matters such as contraception or possible pregnancy, as well as mental health problems such as depressive or suicidal feelings, without other members of their family, especially their parents, knowing about them. This can and indeed often does pose problems when the natural person to see is the family doctor, who also sees other family members. The doctor might maintain confidentiality, but he or she might not, and the uncertainty can and does create acute anxiety. In a survey carried out by the Brook Centre, among girls aged 15–16 years, worries about confidentiality were common. Typical concerns were:

'Doctors are sly … especially if they know your family, you don't know what they'd let slip.' (16-year-old girl)

'It's embarrassing telling your doctor things, 'cos he knows your mum and you think, He's going to be talking to her tomorrow.' (16-year-old girl)

In general, the view of these girls was that doctors were not supposed to tell your parents, but in the end they made their own decision what to do.

'My friend thought she was pregnant and went to the doctors for the Morning After Pill, but he wouldn't give it to her unless she told her mum. But he called and told her in the end.' (16-year-old girl)

'My friend got pregnant, and the doctor called her mum and told her'. (16-year-old girl)

Nurses were not seen as posing as such a threat, because it was thought less likely they would have treated other members of the family, but receptionists were much less trusted.

'Like, supposing you went for a smear test, and the receptionist knew you, they might tell everyone.' (15-year-old girl)

'She's not supposed to tell members of your family if she's friends with them, but she probably will, just through chatting. She's risking her job, but some people are just nosy.' (16-year-old girl)

The needs of young people for advice and help on sexual matters go way beyond guaranteed confidentiality. When, using focus groups, the Brook Centre canvassed the views of young people on what they would like from a sexual health service, they found that a great deal of emphasis was put on the staff being properly trained and competent both in giving contraceptive advice and in counselling. They wanted clinics to be well advertised, accessible, within easy walking distance of a bus stop, and clearly signposted. They wanted clinics to be open five days a week up to 8 pm and Saturday mornings. They hoped that receptionists would be friendly and warm, and treat the young person as an equal, rather than in a patronizing manner. Clinics needed to be pleasantly decorated, secure, and able to ensure privacy. They should be available on a drop-in basis and if it was not possible for a client to be seen within half an hour or so, an offer of an appointment should be made. They should offer a comprehensive service, including dispensing, pregnancy testing, and emotional counselling. Staff should make it clear at the outset that clients do not have to answer questions put to them, and should explain why they are asking any questions that might appear unexpected or surprising. As far as possible, staff should be young or should, at least, convey an attitude sympathetic to the young. They should not make assumptions about a young person's sexuality, so that a gay or lesbian teenager could be treated equally to a heterosexual client.

Now apart from the overriding need for confidentiality, these requirements for a satisfactory service could only emerge from discussions with young people themselves. The focus groups carried out by the Brook make it clear that it is only if young people are regularly consulted about the management of clinics or preferably given some responsibility in management themselves that clinics are likely to be sensitive to their requirements. It is only through empowering young people to speak up and say what they would like that it will become possible to develop a service that meets their needs.

Chapter 7

Alcohol, drugs: having fun or playing with fire?

7.1 How do parents feel about their children drinking alcohol in their teens?

Most parents would find it impossible to give a straight answer to that question. They might perhaps say that they would be very unhappy about their child drinking at 13 years of age, but feel quite relaxed about it by the time their child was at the end of the teens. But the way they behave to their children makes it likely that their attitudes are a great deal more complicated than that would suggest. Many parents who would be horrified if their 13-year-old went to a party where unlimited alcohol was on offer would think it quite normal to let their child have a glass of wine when the family was having a celebratory meal at home. And why not? In contrast, they would probably not feel at all relaxed if their 19-year-old son or daughter was frequently drunk, drinking to relieve feelings of depression, getting into fights while drunk, or having unprotected sex with numerous different partners while drunk. So the answer to the question about how parents feel about their children and alcohol is not straightforward. Clearly the age of the child in question is a major consideration, but so is the amount drunk and the circumstances in which drinking is taking place.

In the years up to the teens, most parents would like to see their children either not drinking alcohol at all, or only drinking in well-supervised situations. Once they reach their teens, parents would like their children to be protected against pressure to make them drink, and well prepared so that by the time they are drinking more and in less well-supervised circumstances, whenever that might be, they are empowered to drink sensibly. The triple requirement for protection, preparation, and empowerment is especially apt when it comes to drink and drugs. I shall contend that if, before their teens, children were much more firmly protected against drinking alcohol unsupervised, and that, once they reached their early or mid-teens, they were empowered to make better choices themselves about their alcohol consumption, there might be a reduction in excessive drinking. In the meantime, if society is serious about wishing to reduce the amount children and young people drink, and adults are prepared to make sacrifices themselves to achieve this aim, this should be quite possible.

7.2 **Alcohol and having fun**

Survey evidence suggests unsurprisingly that most young people in their mid to late teens who drink substantial amounts of alcohol in their teens say they do it to have fun. It makes them feel good. They feel more confident and less inhibited. They find other people more attractive and interesting. Conversation flows more freely. Boys feel more powerful and more virile. It is often said that alcohol increases the desire but reduces the performance. But if a boy cannot bring himself even to talk to a girl unless he has a drink inside him, how he might perform sexually is irrelevant. Girls too feel more at ease in talking to boys after having a drink. They lose some of their worries about being unattractive. They can laugh and flirt less self-consciously.

So do young people in their teens who do not drink alcohol or who drink very little have less fun? That surely depends on what is thought of as fun. If having fun requires a noisy atmosphere, loud laughter, a certain amount of teasing and humiliation, conversation mixed with sexual innuendo and anec-dotes, perhaps followed by sex with a friend or relative stranger, then probably alcohol is a necessary ingredient of the evening's entertainment. On the other hand, if teenagers can also see themselves as having fun if they are talking with their friends, watching a video, going to the cinema, or listening to music, alcohol can seem much less important or perhaps not important at all. Especially if undertaken alone, other activities might be regarded as enjoyable even if not 'fun'. For most teenagers, reading a book or magazine, surfing the 'net', or playing a computer game do not seem to require any alcohol.

When parents are asked what they want for their children in the future, they now often say they don't mind what happens so long as their children are happy. A couple of hundred years ago, very different answers would have been obtained. The risk of ill health or death was so much greater that parents would have, above all, wished for survival of their children into adult life. Now that is taken for granted. The strength of religious feeling in Victorian times would have led many parents living at that time to say that all they wanted for their children was that they should live their lives in the service of God. Such a wish would surely only be that of a tiny minority in western society now. In the middle of the twentieth century, parents might well have said all they wished for their children was that they should 'get on', get a better education than they did, eventually get a better, well-paid job. Such a wish might be seen now as over-ambitious, pushy, wanting one's children to succeed where one has failed oneself. All that is left for parents is to hope their children will be happy.

So children in their teen years who are drinking heavily might say to their parents who are unhappy about how much they are drinking—'Well, you wanted me to be happy and this is what makes me happy, so you should be happy too. It's what you've always wanted for me!' In fact, most young people in their teen years know very well this is not what their parents want. They have the self-control to drink alcohol in moderation and this is what they do.

The idea that it is necessary to drink alcohol to have a good time is one that is strongly promoted by the drinks companies. The marketing directors of these companies know that their best customers are the young. Drinks advertising targets young people in their twenties, often in their early twenties when consumption is at its greatest. There is legislation to prevent advertising directed towards under-age drinkers, but this is not a problem for drinks companies whose marketing staff know that those in their mid-teens wish to imitate young people slightly older than themselves.

In the mid-1990s, drinks companies developed alcopops specifically directed at the youth market. The advertising messages conveyed that these drinks gave you a quick buzz and were risky and exciting. Some of the names they were given made them sound as if they could contain illegal drugs. They were sweet to taste and likely to appeal to those young people who found it difficult to acquire a liking for beer. In fact alcopops were not, in the end, a great marketing success as far as the youth market was concerned, though they have established a modest place for themselves in the drinks market more generally. They were too expensive for most teenagers and never really caught on. But the idea that you need to drink alcohol if you are to have a good time remains a strongly and expensively marketed message that does not just sell brand names, but increases the total alcohol consumption of young people.

It isn't just the drinks companies who promote drinking as the path to happiness. Pubs and wine bars that advertise 'happy hours' are doing just that. Student societies at universities often depend on the financial success of their bars because they are underfunded by their university authorities. So drinking fraternities, such as the tequila club at one well-known London university, subsidize very worthwhile student activities.

7.3 Alcohol, depression, anxiety, and boredom

There is a minority of teenagers who, for a variety of psychological reasons, lack self-control. They may be depressed or unusually anxious and drink to cheer themselves up or to overcome their anxieties. Their depression usually has a number of causes and these were discussed earlier in Chapter 4. But some young people do have biological, perhaps chemical reasons for their depression. More often there is a combination of reasons, both stress and biological vulnerability, that result in depression or overwhelming anxiety. When this happens, teenagers can drown their sorrows in drink just like older people although they are probably a bit less likely to realize what they are doing.

Depression and anxiety are not the only psychological reasons why young people may drink heavily. There are those who have been overactive or hyperactive since early childhood. These often have an unusually powerful need for stimulation. They crave excitement; alcohol may give them just the buzz they feel they need. When hyperactive children are followed up into late adolescence and young adulthood, although most of them drink moderately, they do have higher rates of drink problems than young people who were not hyperactive in earlier childhood.

Finally there are those who have a strong genetic tendency to develop dependence on alcohol. Although no one gene has been definitely identified, it is clear from studies of twins and of the pattern of alcoholism in families that some young people are at great risk of alcohol dependence because of the genes they have inherited, even if they only drink quite moderate amounts to begin with.

7.4 **Peer pressure**

There is a widely held belief that young people in their teens are pressured into drinking by their friends. It is certainly true that young people who drink tend to mix with other young people who do the same. Further, in the drinking scene, competition to down more pints than anyone else or at least to be able to keep up with the quantities others are drinking is important to retain status within the group. But, as American psychologist Dr Ungar suggests, to understand why young people binge drink, it is probably more important to look at why they have joined heavily drinking groups in the first place than to look to pressure from friends. A 15-year-old boy who smokes, who is failing at school, who has parents who themselves smoke and drink heavily, and who, in any case, are too bound up with their own problems to take much notice of him, is much more likely to find himself in a group of friends who drink heavily in or around pubs than to be part of a group that listens to music in different friends' houses or to join a sports club. When he is in a drinking group he may well be spurred on by his mates to drink more, but he wouldn't be at risk of harming himself drinking if he hadn't got into the group in the first place. Like people of any other age, those in their teens mostly choose friends with similar tastes and values.

7.5 **The dark side of drink**

The figures produced in surveys, such as that published each year by John Balding from the Exeter Schools Health Education Unit, giving the numbers of teenagers who drink alcohol and the amount they drink, sound worrying. About one in six 15–16 year old males drink more units than the recommended maximum for adults. However, over half the young people of this age had not consumed any alcohol at all in the pervious week. In another survey, a quarter of British 15–16-year-olds said they had been binge-drinking three or more times in the last 30 days. Many young people who get drunk damage property and a greater number get into arguments and fights. Reliable figures for even more serious effects of alcohol are not available in Britain, but in the USA most fatal car crashes involving teenagers are at least partly caused by alcohol. Those young people who commit suicide more often than not have been drinking heavily. Murderers and murder victims are commonly suffering from the effects of alcohol. Alcohol is partly responsible for the three most common causes of death in adolescence in the United States (automobile accidents, homicide, and suicide) and for the two most common causes (automobile accidents and suicide) in Britain.

There are other worrying effects of excessive drinking. Each year about a thousand young people in their teens or even younger are admitted to hospital Accident and Emergency (A. and E.) Departments, comatose and unrousable, with acute alcohol poisoning. It is unusual for young people to commit crimes so that they can obtain money for drink. Instead it is the disinhibiting effects of alcohol on the individual that lead to fights and damaging property.

As the 1995 Royal College of Physicians Report makes clear, the link between youth crime as well as other forms of antisocial behaviour and alcohol is well established and strong. A working party on 'Young People and Alcohol' convened by the Home Office Standing Conference on Crime Prevention concluded that alcohol was a common cause of youth crime, particularly crimes involving violence. This working party cited evidence that '50% of a sample of victims of wounding reported that the offender had been drinking, as did 44% of victims of common assault and 30% of victims of sexual offences'. It has been suggested that this gives a false picture of the link between alcohol and violence because, for some violent individuals, having had too much to drink is a habitual state and that therefore one would expect a high proportion of violent offences to be committed by people in this state, even though alcohol was not responsible for their violence. This view seems to offend against common sense and is contrary to the almost universal experience that alcohol removes inhibitions that stop young people being aggressive.

There are other problems unrelated to crime. It is not at all unusual for older school pupils to go to school with a hangover that affects their concentration. About one in five exclusions from school occur because of drinking alcohol on school premises. It is common for university students to be unable to follow a morning lecture because they are hung over from the night before. Some, at least, of the vast debts that many students build up while they are at university can be put down to purchase of alcohol.

There are also strong links in teenagers and young adults between alcohol and unsafe sex. Around two in five 13- and 14-year-olds were 'drunk or stoned' when they first experienced sexual intercourse. The same proportion of 16–24-year-olds say they are more likely to have casual sex after drinking. About 20% of young men and women admit to having unsafe sex after drinking too much, and it seems highly likely that the rates are higher in those in their teens.

Alcohol consumption is increasing among the young. Among 11–15-year-olds, mean weekly consumption rose from 5.3 units in 1990 to 9.9 units in 1998. That means that in 1998 the average 13-year-old drank on average half a pint of beer a day. In fact, most drank their weekly amounts in one or two sessions of 4 pints or so at the weekend. These levels of alcohol consumption in children and young people in Britain are mirrored in some other European countries, particularly Denmark, Poland, and Ireland, but, as the 1999 European school survey reports, in many other European countries a reverse trend is occurring. In particular, in France and Italy, alcohol consumption is falling, though admittedly from very high levels. It is not at all clear why there should be these differences between countries, but there is no doubt they exist. French university students may drink one or two beers in the evening with friends, but, though of course there are exceptions, they do not drink to get drunk to anything like the extent of British students.

Alcohol dependence, the inability to have one drink without going on to get drunk, although unusual in adolescence, is common in young people in their twenties and thirties. It nearly always begins with heavy drinking in adolescence. It is responsible for many more deaths in adult life than drugs. In Britain, there are approximately 30 000 deaths attributable to alcohol each year, compared to around 500 deaths from illicit drugs.

There is a more cheerful statistic concerning teen drinking. Most adolescents who are heavy drinkers do not go on to become dependent on alcohol. They mainly reduce their intake when they reach their late teens or early twenties, start getting serious about their careers, and live together with a partner or at least have a stable relationship. It isn't possible to predict with any accuracy which heavy teen drinkers are likely to go on to develop dependence on alcohol.

In general, those who are at greatest risk are the heaviest drinkers, those who have other members of their family who are alcohol dependent, those who drink for psychological reasons (such as depression, anxiety, or seeking excitement), those who are also on illegal drugs and smoke, and those who are unable to find jobs or make stable relationships.

7.6 **What can parents do if they *really* want to reduce their child's alcohol intake?**

Nick is a 15-year-old living in a village on the Welsh borders. He has been drinking alcohol and smoking since he was ten, and his alcohol consumption has recently gone up considerably. It is not surprising that he drinks heavily, as his father has had treatment for alcoholism, and his mother drinks quite heavily too. He has recently got in with a group of young men, aged between 16 and 23 years, who meet in the centre of the village at 8 pm every Friday and get into a minibus driven by a 50-year-old teetotaller who is paid well to drive them into the big city 20 miles away. They drink until about 11 pm in a pub and then emerge if not looking for a fight, at least prepared to get involved if one arises. Although he has only been in the group 6 weeks, Nick has already had to go twice to an Accident and Emergency Department to have his hand and face stitched up and once to a Police Station to be charged with causing an affray. How should his parents react? More pointedly, in view of their own lifestyle, how can they react?

In contrast to their reactions if they discover their teenage children are using illegal drugs, many parents think it is rather funny when their children come home drunk for the first time. This is especially likely if they are heavy drinkers themselves. Now one episode of drunkenness is certainly no cause for panic. Indeed parental panic will probably do more harm than good. But it probably isn't helpful to pass off episodes of drunkenness as trivial. Certainly if teenage children start to come home drunk every Saturday night, if there are signs their schoolwork is being affected by drinking, if they are in trouble for getting into fights or for damaging property, then there is a real cause for concern.

Parents who are concerned about the amount their children are drinking will find it easier to deal with the matter if they start off with a relationship with them that permits conversation about difficult topics. This is more likely to exist (see Chapter 3) if parents have got into the habit of listening to their children, talking with them rather than at them, trying not to be shocked by what they are told, explaining their own feelings, noticing when their children are upset or anxious, and taking their feelings seriously.

Parents can help to cut down the risks if they encourage their teenage children to stick to lower-strength brands and not to drink too quickly. This will not be easy if their child is in a group where the whole point of drinking is to get drunk as cheaply and as quickly as possible. Their children will probably already be aware of the dangers of being given spiked drinks and of spiking someone else's drink. It is important to agree rules on parties held in their own home even if there may not be all that much they can do about parties held elsewhere. Removing their own stock of drink, especially spirits, is a sensible precaution for parents to take. Providing plenty to eat will at least make sure that drink is not consumed on an empty stomach. For parties away from home it is helpful to make sure there is a way of getting home safely when it is over.

Most young people in their teen years drink sensibly. They may binge occasionally, but mostly they keep their drinking under control. A significant minority do not and some of these will get into real trouble.

What can parents do if their children are frequently coming home drunk, getting into fights when drunk, not getting up in the morning because they are hung over or getting into debt as a result of drinking? As far as possible it is helpful if parents make clear what their feelings are about the situation, but make clear they are still fond of their children and will try to stick with them. Nearly all young people in their teens who are drinking heavily will be earning money in a part-time job to finance their consumption. If their generous pocket money allowance is going straight into the pub till, parents may feel they want to keep control of the situation by reducing it. Encouraging young people to go to the doctor to talk about excessive drinking is a thankless task. Most don't see their drinking as a health problem. On the other hand, if they have other problems such as depression or overwhelming anxiety, they may be prepared to go to a counsellor or even to their doctor to discuss the situation. This may result in referral to a specialist drug and alcohol action team where there will be people skilled in improving the motivation of young people to accept help. And once a young person has accepted the need for help, the process of rehabilitation is much smoother.

7.7 **What if we, as a society, *really* wanted to reduce alcohol consumption?**

The above account of how much parents can do to limit the amount their teen children drink has revealed the limitations of parental influence. Frankly, in a social climate that encourages the consumption of alcohol as a sign of adulthood and as a necessary accompaniment to most forms of enjoyment, parents stand little chance of success. Yet the increase in alcohol consumption over the years in Britain and the fact that consumption varies so much from country to country should encourage us to believe that moderate drinking ought to be a realistic target for social policy. If social factors have led to a rise in alcohol consumption, surely social change could result in a corresponding fall. Certainly we cannot blame the genes. The young in Britain today have the same genes as those who lived half a century ago, and an identical gene pattern to those in other western countries. So there is nothing genetic about the changes in alcohol consumption.

In what ways might society change to achieve more moderate alcohol consumption in the young? The possibilities seem to be limited to three approaches: changes in the law, in education, and in taxation. None of these is likely to make any difference at all before one delicate issue has been tackled. Consumption in the young very closely mirrors that in older people. Unless consumption in older people drops it is most unlikely that there will be any change in consumption by the young. So society has to decide whether it is prepared to contemplate measures that will affect, perhaps even limit the freedom of the whole population merely for the protection of the young. Perhaps it is not, but let us pursue this possibility and, bearing in mind the triple need to protect, prepare, and empower, see if it leads to any acceptable policies.

7.8 Changes in the law

At the present time, the law relating to underage drinking is in a mess, partly because it is so complicated. Legally, a parent or any other person may not give alcohol to a child under five except on medical orders. Between five and sixteen years a child may consume alcohol at home. They may not buy or be bought a drink in a pub or licensed premises until the age of 18 years, unless they are over 16 years when they can buy or be bought cider or beer if part of a meal. Up to 14 years they can however go into a pub, provided it is not part of the pub where alcohol is both sold and drunk. The 14- and 15-year-olds can go anywhere in a pub, but cannot drink alcohol there. At 18 years, but not before, a young person may buy and drink alcohol in a bar and can buy alcohol in an off-licence, including a supermarket.

The law is frequently broken. In particular, from about the age of 14 years it is relatively easy in most parts of the country for 'under age' young people to buy alcohol in off-licence premises. Reasonably mature looking young people also have little problem in buying and consuming alcohol in pubs. Young people under the age of 16 years can also often succeed in giving money to adults and persuading them to buy alcohol for them in off-licences.

Various measures have been recommended or are in place to reduce illegal sales and the consumption of alcohol by young people. All forms of sales promotion towards the young are subject to regulation. The marketing of alcohol that might specifically appeal to children and young people is against the law, and there is a voluntary code of practice monitored for infringements of this code by the Portman Group, an organization financed by the drinks industry. There is encouragement to landlords and those owning off-licenses to demand proof of age when selling alcohol to people who might be underage. These measures seem to have had no effect at all on the consumption of alcohol by children and young people. This continues to rise year by year. Young people get a great deal of pleasure out of drinking alcohol and the increase in consumption would not matter if the harmful effects were not so serious.

The inadequacy of existing legislation to influence the situation is illustrated by the statistics on alcohol consumption by the young. This increases in a steady manner year by year from about the age of 14 years onwards to reach a peak at around the age of 22–23 years after which it declines. If the legislation made any significant difference one would expect a slow increase from 14 to 18 years and then a sharp increase at 18 years when buying alcohol in pubs and off-licenses becomes legal. This just does not occur.

All the same, even though British laws seem to make little impact, it would be wrong to say that there is no evidence that changes in the law could never make a difference. For example, Michael Windle has described how, in the United States, a number of states have enacted legislation (Minimum Legal Drinking Age—MLDA), making it an offence for an under 21-year-old to purchase alcohol. Despite the fact that it is clear that this law is regularly flouted (George W. Bush's daughters are far from being the only under 21-year-olds to have done so), it has made a difference. A number of studies have been carried out on its effects by comparing states with and without MLDA. It is reasonably clear that such legislation results in small reductions in consumption not just in the under 21s, but even up to the age of 25. More striking is the reduction in traffic crashes among young people. In some states reductions of around 15% have been recorded. Further, Windle reports, alcohol-related traffic deaths have reduced in the same states by 59%, from 5380 in 1982 to 2201 in 1995.

Another piece of legislation enacted in some of the United States but not in others that seems to have made a difference is that concerned with the blood alcohol concentration (BAC) alcohol permitted to drivers under the age of 21 years. In the UK, the permitted BAC level is 80 mg%. In some of the United States this has been reduced to 20 mg%, an amount so small that it is virtually a ban on any alcoholic consumption before driving. In the States where this law is in force, this has resulted in a 20% reduction in night-time, single driver fatal crashes in 15–20-year-olds. This legal measure has also been effective in other countries such as Australia, where, in some states it has been supplemented by random breath tests, not just in the young, but across the whole age range. This policy resulted in a 36% decline in alcohol-involved traffic crashes.

Where does this evidence lead to in terms of desirable changes in legislation in Britain and in other countries with similar legislation? Although the MLDA legislation in the USA might suggest it would be a good idea to introduce it in other countries, it is by no means certain it would be effective elsewhere. American youth are more often in employment and have more disposable income than those in other countries. Alcoholic drinks are cheaper there than elsewhere. Many more of them own their own cars or have access to cars. Further, MLDA is age discriminatory. While it can be seen and doubtless is widely seen as protective of young people, it takes away the rights of young people highly competent to make up their own minds how much they want to drink.

In contrast, there are many attractions to the introduction of legislation relating to a reduced BAC across the board and which is not just limited to the young. After all, drivers of any age who are incompetent because of alcohol consumption are a menace to other people. It is true that under 21s are at highest risk for causing accidents, but, because there are far more of them and they drive more, most accidents are caused by people who are over that age. Disqualification from driving for people of all ages found to have a BAC over 20 mg% would be protective of other drivers and, incidentally, pedestrians.

A more radical suggestion is to abolish all existing underage legislation and replace it with a blanket ban on drinking alcohol by under 14-year-olds in pubs or other public places, but allowing those over this age to drink alcohol if they want to. This is precisely what young people over the age of 14 years are doing at the present time, despite a mass of poorly thought out, futile legislation aimed to prevent them from doing so. If instead of trying to stop them drinking there were greater sanctions on inflicting injury on others with higher fines and longer community sentences with rehabilitation and education for those found to have a BAC over 20 mg%, whatever their age, this could well have a deterrent effect both on excessive alcohol consumption and on violent crime. Better still, one might look to ways of rewarding drivers who don't drink, perhaps by offering lower insurance premiums to those in this category, though, of course, the insurance companies would not pay up, except on a third party basis, if an accident occurred and there was evidence that alcohol had been consumed. There are parallels with life insurance premiums and smoking as well as with car insurance companies and accidents when drivers and passengers are not wearing seat belts.

7.9 **Education**

The first thing to say about educational measures to reduce drinking in the young by concentrating on the young is that they are a great disappointment. It is the right of young people to be given information about alcohol and its effects, so this statement by no means entails a suggestion that alcohol education in school is a waste of time. But all the attempts to show that education in school can change drinking *behaviour* to a significant extent have failed. Lectures are a complete waste of time if one is trying to change behaviour. On the other hand, there is reasonably good evidence that lessons that are more interactive and involve teaching skills in refusing drinks when offered do have a small, but definite effect in reducing alcohol consumption. There is little evidence though that this effect is anything but short-term, and therefore while not completely useless, it has very limited value.

One might expect education in school that is linked to similar education in the family and in the community to be more likely to have an impact. This would make sense. If messages in school are countered by exactly opposite messages learned in the family and from the media, one can hardly expect them to hit home. So it is perhaps surprising that those extremely expensive American programmes that target schools, parents, the media, and community leaders at the same time have also had a very small and disappointing effect on alcohol consumption in the young. (Results are distinctly more positive when it comes to drugs and I shall discuss this later on.) Perhaps this gives the answer to the question whether the whole population is prepared to modify its behaviour for the benefit of the young. The answer seems to be in the negative if an educational approach alone is employed.

7.10 **Taxation**

There is really good evidence from a number of studies, carried out in different countries, and described by Griffiths Edwards and his colleagues, that the higher the tax on alcohol, the lower the consumption. Further, the young are particularly price sensitive when it comes to alcohol, so the effect of taxation is greater on them than it is on the rest of the population. It has been estimated in the United States that a rise of 10 cents in the cost of a beer might be expected to reduce alcohol consumption in the young by 11%. A fall in price in distilled spirits has been shown to result in a rise in consumption in the general population in Finland, Italy, and Kenya. Rises in the price of beer and wine have been shown to result in a relative decline in alcohol consumption in the whole population in the UK, Sweden, Germany, and Belgium. In fact, in the UK, the Chancellor of the Exchequer has much greater influence over the amount of alcohol consumption in the young than the Secretaries of State for Health and Trade and Industry combined. Once again we have to ask ourselves whether the adult population is prepared to suffer higher prices for alcohol for the benefit of the young. This is a particularly important issue for Britain, that is quite likely to be exposed to pressure to reduce its alcohol taxation to bring it into line with the rest of Europe. Sadly, the answer may depend on whether decisions are taken near an election.

7.11 Drugs and alcohol: the similarities

Everyone knows that alcohol is, in fact, a drug. Yet everyone also knows that when we talk about drugs and young people we do not mean alcohol, but among other substances, cannabis, amphetamine, ecstasy, magic mushrooms, heroin, and cocaine. That is how I shall use the word 'drug' in this chapter.

All the same, it is worth emphasizing that separating illegal drugs like those I have mentioned from alcohol and indeed, from nicotine, is, in most ways, by no means logical. They are all used, smoked, drunk, eaten, injected, inhaled, consumed, or whatever for their pleasurable psychological effects. Their use always has a symbolic importance as a sign of having made it to adulthood. They are all social lubricants, making it easier for people, especially for shy young people, to socialize because they are sharing an enjoyable experience in common. They all have harmful side effects. Different people react differently to the same substance, whatever it may be. One can become addicted to alcohol and nicotine just as one can to illegal drugs.

There are indeed so many similarities between drugs and alcohol it is not at all surprising that, when drugs, though illegal, are easily available, as they are in many parts of Britain, young people in their teens feel free to choose between them and alcohol when they are planning how to spend an evening out. So if they do not want their parents to know what they have been up to, they may decide alcohol is likely to be more easily detectable on the breath when they return home and choose drugs. If they want to spend an evening listening to dreamy music with friends, they may again prefer drugs. If they like the idea of a noisy evening in a pub, perhaps with the prospect of a scrap afterwards, they will go for alcohol. If they are planning a sexual experience and feel the need to get tanked up before getting up the courage to 'pull' a partner for the evening or night, alcohol may again be the choice. On the other hand, if they already have a sexual partner in mind, and want to be at their maximum sexual performance, they may avoid alcohol and go for drugs. If they want a feeling of excitement and energy at a late night or an all night club, they may choose a mixture of alcohol and a stimulant drug such as ecstasy or amphetamine. Finally, they may be hugely influenced by the cost of these different substances. Especially in early and mid-teen age, they are quite likely to go for the cheapest alternative.

7.12 **Drugs and alcohol: the differences**

There are, of course, massive differences in the effects different drugs and alcohol have, in the health risks their use involves, and in how the law regards them. To make this clear, it is necessary to give a brief account of those most commonly taken. (What follows is taken from the Health Education Council Guide for Parents and the Royal College of Psychiatrists Report.) Incidentally, although some of the more enduring slang names for these drugs are given, these change virtually by the month, so it is just not possible for a book like this to provide an up-to-date list.

Amphetamine (also known as Speed, Whizz, Uppers, and Amph). This is taken as a grey or white powder that is snorted, swallowed, injected, or dissolved as a drink, or in tablets that are swallowed. It is taken for the feeling of excitement and heightened alertness it gives. After its use, young people may feel tired and depressed for a day or two, and the use of high doses may bring about acute panic and hallucinations. Long-term use puts a strain on the heart and may cause mental illness. Addiction is not common, but does occur. There are about 10 deaths a year in the UK from this drug.

Cannabis (also known as marijuana, weed, shit, hash, spliff). This is usually smoked in a spliff or joint, which is rolled, often mixed with tobacco, though it can also be eaten in various forms, including a 'cake'. It produces a pleasurable feeling of dreamy relaxation and detachment. 'Stoned' is a term usually used to describe this state. After smoking it, users often feel tired and may lack motivation for hours or even days afterwards. It impairs the ability to concentrate and to learn. Driving may be adversely affected. Probably only partly because it is often mixed with tobacco, it increases the risk of lung cancer. Dependence on cannabis is unusual with those who only use the drug at weekends, though it does occur. It is quite common among daily users. If dependency occurs, withdrawal is unpleasant but usually not as difficult as it is with other drugs. Some people think that heavy use is also followed by a chronic lack of motivation and drive. It is uncertain how many deaths a year occur as a result of using cannabis, but, excluding the uncertain deaths from lung cancer linked to habitual use, the number is probably very small.

Magic Mushrooms (also known as 'shrooms' or 'mushies'). These are usually eaten raw, dried, or cooked. They change the way surroundings are perceived, for example making colours and sounds distorted, with the sense of movement speeded up or slowed down. The experience is known as a 'trip'. Magic mushrooms can cause intestinal symptoms, especially diarrhoea. There is a serious possibility of eating poisonous mushrooms by mistake resulting in serious illness or even death.

LSD (otherwise known as acid, or trips). This is usually eaten in small squares of paper with a picture on one side. It may also be taken in 'dots' or tiny tablets. It has the same effects as magic mushrooms, but the perceptual distortions are much more intense. LSD users may find themselves on a terrifyingly bad 'trip', they cannot stop. Afterwards they may experience uncontrollable flashbacks to a previous bad 'trip'. LSD can make existing mental illness worse. The number of deaths a year is not known, but is probably very small.

Heroin (otherwise known as smack, gear, junk, and scag). This is consumed as a brownish-white powder that is dissolved and injected, smoked, or snorted. It gives the user a sense of warmth and well-being or, in larger doses, produces feelings of drowsiness and relaxation. It is highly addictive and repeated use for 2–3 weeks leads to tolerance, the user needing much larger amounts of the drug to produce the same effect. Addicts require the drug to give them a 'rush' of intense pleasure as well as to avoid extremely unpleasant withdrawal symptoms. Sharing needles leads to a high risk of contracting an infection, especially Hepatitis B or C, or an HIV infection followed by AIDS and death. There are about 200 deaths a year from heroin use, but a much larger number of young people have their lives destroyed by this drug.

Cocaine and Crack (also known as coke, Charlie, C, and snow). This is taken as a white powder snorted up the nose, or is sometimes dissolved and injected. Crack is smoked by playing a flame on a small crystal and directly inhaling the smoke containing the vapour. Cocaine and crack give a sense of well-being, alertness, and confidence. The effect lasts about 30 min and users are left craving for more. Users then 'crash', feeling exhausted, anxious, and hungry. Both cocaine and crack are highly addictive and craving can last for months after the last use. Snorting can produce damage to the inside of the nose, as well as heart problems, and sometimes severe mental symptoms. The number of deaths from cocaine or crack cocaine a year is unknown, as is the number whose lives are ruined by it.

Ecstasy (also known as E, disco biscuits, and fantasy). This comes in tablets of different sizes, shapes, and colour. The drug gives a sense of energy, alertness, and arousal. Sound, colour, and emotions seem more intense. These effects last from 3 to 6 hours. Use can lead to tiredness and depression for days afterwards. There is a risk of overheating and dehydration leading to collapse or even death. However, over-enthusiastic drinking of vast quantities of fluid can also be dangerous. The drug has been reported to cause changes in the brains of experimental animals. The drug causes about 10 deaths a year, but the number may be rising.

Glues and aerosols. These are inhaled from products such as lighter gas refills, hairspray, deodorant or air freshener aerosols, tins or tubes of glue, paints and paint thinners. They are usually inhaled from a piece of cloth or sleeve, but gas products may be squirted directly into the back of the throat. Users feel drunk, dizzy, giggly, and dreamy. They may develop hallucinations. Vomiting, blackouts, and heart problems may occur. There is a risk of suffocation if the product is inhaled from a plastic bag over the head. Long-term use may damage the brain, liver, and kidneys. There are about 100 deaths a year from solvent abuse and the number may be rising.

Tranquillizers (mostly from the group of drugs known as benzodiazepines, especially temazepam and diazepam, trade name—valium). These may be legally prescribed or bought illegally. They are in the form of tablets that can be swallowed. They used to be produced in capsule form, but the liquid in the capsules was used for injection, so capsule production was halted and this has probably markedly reduced the practice. They are used mainly to reduce anxiety and tension and create a feeling of calm. They can be addictive and users may find it difficult to wean themselves off the tablets because of panic attacks.

The effects of these drugs is therefore greatly variable. But their effects have one important common element. They virtually all give an immediate sense of well being and pleasure, followed after anything from a few minutes to a few hours by feelings of emptiness, sadness, and at least a wish, sometimes a craving for a repeat dose. Those who have tried to measure the balance of pleasure and mental pain linked to drug use have nearly all concluded that, except perhaps for low dose cannabis use, pain outweighs pleasure. Sadly drug use rarely occurs after a cold calculation of the benefits and costs. If it did, there would be many fewer drugs consumed.

As with alcohol, the legal status of illegal drugs is complicated. In the UK, the Misuse of Drugs Act divides illegal drugs into three groups. *Class A* includes amphetamines if prepared for injection, cocaine and crack cocaine, ecstasy, heroin, LSD, and magic mushrooms. The maximum penalty for possession is seven years prison and a fine. Possession with an intent to supply may result in life imprisonment and/or a fine. *Class B* drugs include amphetamines as tablets and cannabis. The maximum penalty for possession is five years prison and/or a fine. Possession with an intent to supply can lead to a maximum of 14 years in prison and/or a fine. *Class C* drugs include the benzodiazepines, such as temazepam and valium. Illegal possession can lead to a maximum of two years in prison and/or a fine. Possession with an intent to supply can result in five years in prison and/or a fine.

At the time of writing (Autumn 2003) there are strong indications that the UK Government intends to reclassify cannabis as a Class C drug.

7.13 Drugs and crime

As a Royal College of Psychiatrists report published in the year 2000 makes clear, the links between drugs and crime are complicated. Some young offenders steal or break into property, something they have never done before, to fund a lifestyle that includes drug use. Others have been offenders before they become involved in heavy drug use, which amplifies a crime career. Most young people who use less costly drugs such as cannabis, ecstasy, or amphetamines just at weekends or less often are often spending no more than they would on alcohol, so one wouldn't expect them to be pushed into criminality to acquire extra funds. But heavy use of cocaine or heroin is much more expensive, with daily use of heroin or cocaine costing around £40–£75 a day. It has been suggested that if one includes possessing drugs and supplying them, around half of all recorded crime includes a drug-related element. Among problem drug users, of whom only a minority are still in their teens, imprisonment is common and over 50% of injecting drug users have been in prison at some time. Young girls who are prostitutes have often been forced into prostitution in order to pay for otherwise unaffordable drugs.

7.14 Young people and drugs in Britain and elsewhere

The good news is that the great majority of children and young people in Britain are not using drugs in a way that puts their health at risk. It is true that a high proportion of young people are smoking cannabis. This is true for over a third from the age of 16 years onwards. It is also true that cannabis can harm health and that young people are particularly likely to develop dependence on it. It is also the case that the UK has higher rates of cannabis use than any other European country apart from France. All this is true, but the facts are that most of those who smoked the drug did so either just to see what it was like and either never or hardly again, or settled down to occasional use mostly at the weekends. There is little evidence that, used moderately like this, cannabis is bad for health or causes dependency. So it is probably true to say that over 90% or more of Britain's children and young people are not putting their health at risk because of cannabis. Further, survey evidence suggests that the numbers of young people using cannabis went down slightly in the second half of the 1990s so, in so far as cannabis use is a problem, it is not getting worse.

A similar picture can be drawn for the use of ecstasy. Although the frequency of use of this drug went up considerably in the 1990s and continues to go up in the first years of the twenty-first century, the great majority of young people at least in their mid-teens do not use it and, of those who do, most do not suffer harm as a result. Just over 3%, or around one in 30 British 15–16-year-olds reported using ecstasy in the 1999 European Survey and there have been either no deaths or a very tiny number of deaths of young people of this age arising from the use of ecstasy.

This good news does not mean that all parents of young people in their teens can be reassured that their children are at very low or no risk from the use of drugs. For a relatively small minority of parents the news is very far from good; indeed it is horrifying. A low but increasing number of young people under the age of 18 years are using the highly addictive drugs, heroin and cocaine. Solvent abuse or glue sniffing remains widespread, especially in younger children aged around 9–15 years and, as we have seen, causes around 75–100 deaths a year in the UK.

Young people at risk of addiction to heroin and cocaine or glue sniffing are not a random selection of the child and adolescent population. Far from it. They are likely to be living on run-down estates in deprived areas where trading in drugs is widespread. Even within such neighbourhoods, who does and who does not become addicted is, to a considerable degree, predictable. Children whose parents can keep an eye on their whereabouts (and this will be easier where there are two parents rather than one), living in homes where relationships are marked by affection and harmony, who are going to school regularly and doing reasonably well there, who are able to concentrate on tasks and who do not crave excitement, who do not smoke cigarettes, who participate in sports, hobbies, or other leisure activities, who do not have other family members using drugs, and who have friends who do not use drugs, are at relatively low risk even if they are living in very disadvantaged circumstances. Those who do not enjoy these advantages are at higher risk, and the more of these advantages they lack, the more at risk they are.

Brian is a 15-year-old boy living with both his parents in a middle class area on the outskirts of Birmingham. He is doing well at school and is predicted to get good grades in public examinations. He has numerous friends and two best friends. He gets on well with his parents and his younger sister. A year ago, when he was round at a friend's house, one of his group produced some cannabis and they shared several joints. Brian had previously smoked a few cigarettes, but his parents had found out and had been so upset, he had decided not to smoke any more. The joints made him feel pretty good and relaxed, but he also felt sick after them. He and his friends continued to share joints at weekends over the next few months, but the boy who supplied them left the area and his group made no attempt to get any more. Brian's parents do not know that he has used cannabis and would be horrified if they did. However, he can hardly be classed as an 'experimental' user as he used the drug over quite a long period. Brian kept very quiet when drugs were discussed in class and did not disagree with the teacher giving the class even when, from his own experience, he knew that some of the information provided was wrong.

Sam is a 15-year-old boy living on a Council Estate with his mother and stepfather. He gets on well with his mother, but has a terrible relationship with his stepfather, with whom he has had several physical fights. His attendance at school, where he is supposed to be in a remedial stream, is fitful and he can only read at about a nine-year level. His older brother has been on several drugs charges, both for possessing heroin and, on one occasion resulting in a two-year prison sentence, for selling it. Sam has smoked cigarettes since he was nine years old and now smokes 20 a day. He has never smoked cannabis, but was introduced to heroin injection at the age of 14 years by a friend of his brother. He now needs to find around £50 a day to fund his drug habit, which he does without too much difficulty by shoplifting, occasional drug trading, and some housebreaking. He has made four or five attempts to wean himself off drugs, but has never lasted more than a few hours. Now he is in a poor physical state and is constantly angry and depressed.

7.15 **What parents can do about drugs**

The stories of Brian and Sam make it clear that helping children to avoid harming themselves with drugs has to begin in early childhood. Those children who, when first faced with drugs, have previously received affection and warmth, have good friends who are not themselves in trouble, and enjoy learning at school will have a low chance of being harmed by drugs. Previous positive experiences at home and school are by no means a complete guarantee against harm from drugs, but they are a pretty sound protection. Given the lack of any effective means of controlling the supply of dangerous, illegal drugs, trying to ensure that the young have high self-esteem, value themselves, and think they have a worthwhile future is, in fact, the only effective means of protecting them.

There are also more specific ways parents can help. They can try to make sure that, before they are faced with drugs, their children have some essential information about them. It is better if this is realistic information, and does not exaggerate the dangers. Some parents might think that if you can die from drugs, it is surely hardly possible to exaggerate the dangers, but children will rapidly realize this is a fate of only a tiny minority of those who take drugs. If parents exaggerate, they are more likely to be ignored altogether. But children do need to know that *all* drugs can have harmful effects, they can all be dangerous for some people, it is dangerous to mix drugs, and pretty well all drugs they buy are likely to be impure and mixed with other substances. They also need to know that if they ever get as far as injecting drugs (and they shouldn't), sharing syringes carries a great risk of becoming infected with one of a number of fatal diseases.

Many parents find it so difficult to discuss drugs with their children, they avoid it and trust to teachers to do this. But it does make a difference for children to be able to talk to their parents about drugs. Parents may find it less hard if they show their main concern is for their children's health, safety, and well-being, if they listen carefully to what their children say and feel, explaining their own views as honestly and openly as they can. Preaching and threats work less well than listening and explaining.

It is helpful for parents to be able to recognize signs of drug taking. Changes in appearance or in eating and sleeping habits, secretiveness, and moodiness may be indications, but they are more likely to be due to trouble with friends or to being in love. Of course, if parents find quantities of empty glue cans or smell chemicals on the breath, they can be pretty sure their children are sniffing solvents. Most parents will be able to recognize the stale grassy smell of cannabis. Finding tablets or syringes will probably only be a confirmation of what parents have suspected for some time.

If parents are pretty sure their children are taking drugs, it is usually not helpful to avoid raising the subject. Parents might try to find a time when they can discuss the situation without interruptions. They might begin by asking how their child feels generally and then confess, without accusations, they have been worried about their child using drugs. Accusations usually just lead to arguments. Those in their teens need the opportunity to express their feelings. They will often deny they are using drugs and, if they admit it, will often say they have the situation under control and their parents are not to worry. If at all possible, parents should try to leave the lines of communication with their children open.

If they are concerned their child is becoming a habitual user and harming health in this way, parents will usually want to encourage their child to get advice from a Drugs Helpline (numbers are given at the end of the book). If their children don't want to do this, parents may find it helpful to contact the helpline themselves to get advice on their own behalf. Drug Action Teams now exist in every area and, although they may be under-staffed, they do have effective means of treatment for motivated young people available to them. Parents are likely to feel desperate if their child becomes drug-dependent. Again they should try and get help by talking to professionals and other people in similar situations (try the Families Anonymous HelpLine).

7.16 **What society could do about drugs**

Children and young people are not often discussed when questions relating to drugs are raised. It is assumed, for example, that if drugs were legalized, this would have little impact on consumption by children, because it would be easy to control the sale of drugs to children under the age of 18. The degree to which alcohol is sold to young people despite clear legislation outlawing the practice, suggests it would be far from easy.

Our attitudes to drug use both generally and in those in their teens in particular, might be clarified if we look more broadly at the way we try to find means both to protect young people and to ensure they have the skills they need to protect themselves. There is a very large number of enjoyable, legal activities in which those in their teens engage that are significantly risky. They include cycling (especially in the city), rock climbing, white water rafting, canoeing, and playing rugby. Every year a very small number of young people in their teens are killed or seriously maimed while engaged in such activities. How are these activities different from drug use, which, at least as far as cannabis and ecstasy are concerned, are also enjoyable to those engaged in them, but risky and the cause of very small numbers of deaths and brain injury? Could we develop a set of principles that might apply to all such activities?

A first principle might be that the young should be firmly protected from engaging in significantly risky activities until they are themselves capable of appraising the risks. Parents should surely be discouraged from letting their children engage in significantly risky activities just because they think their children will find them enjoyable. Parents do have to be allowed to put their children at risk in some unavoidable circumstances. These include necessary surgical operations, or even exposing them to immunizations with a very low risk when the risk of not being immunized is greater.

Second, before they engage in significantly risky activities, children should be well prepared for them so that risk of harm is minimized.

Third, when developing policies for commercial promotion of significantly risky activities, a distinction should be drawn between those that carry risk of long-term harm and those that only carry risk when they are undertaken. Cigarette smoking and drug use are examples of the former, cycling and canoeing of the latter. Commercial promotion to the young of activities carrying risk of long-term harm should be banned. Because the young are exposed to and influenced by advertisement meant for adults, this means that such advertisement should be banned completely. Trading in these activities should be strictly regulated. But, above all, education for those who wish to resist involvement in such activities should be universally available. And those who do not wish to resist need an honest and open discussion of the risks they are taking.

Drugs education in schools presents special problems not shared by alcohol or sex education. When teachers teach about drugs they are, at the present time, teaching about a crime on the statute books. Nowadays teachers are encouraged to put over the message that it is better not to take drugs at all, but those who do should try to limit the harm they do to themselves. 'Harm limitation' is replacing 'Just say no to drugs' as the message to get over.

This seems very sensible, but there is a catch. Suppose the crime in question were not taking drugs but taking and driving away cars. Would society tolerate a situation where classroom teaching involved imparting the idea to children that it is better not to steal other people's cars, but adding information for those impelled to take and drive away how to get into a locked car without causing too much damage and then how to drive it without having an accident? Surely not. Encouraging 'harm limitation' in the use of drugs in an open and honest way, surely a desirable activity in a society in which such harmful substances are so widely consumed, is only possible where consumption is not illegal.

There are various ways in which the use of drugs might be decriminalized. These range from reclassifying cannabis from Class B to Class C, changes in policing to stop charging for possession of cannabis for personal use, and changes in legalization to decriminalize and possibly legalize first the less harmful drugs and then those that are more addictive. There are arguments for and against all of these. They involve the cost and effectiveness of control, the likely increase or decrease in usage if change was brought about, and the impact on the rate of violent crime if obtaining and possessing small amounts of less harmful drugs was no longer an offence.

When the impact of these possible changes on the lives of young people in their teens is considered, the situation is not at all straightforward, but, with young people in mind, there seem to me to be impelling reasons for some degree of liberalization in relation to the less harmful drugs. First, the purchase of less harmful illegal drugs brings young people into contact with those peddling much more harmful substances. Second, the cost of ineffective control is vast. If control costs were cut, more police time could be spent controlling the supply of more harmful drugs and more money could be spent on services for those who were drug-dependent or at risk of dependency. More could also be spent on preventing drug usage in those in their very early teens and younger who are not in a position to make informed choices for themselves. Third, as I have already suggested, the education of the young would be easier for both teachers and parents if the decriminalization of less harmful drugs occurred.

We have some evidence from other countries that some cautious degree of liberalization does not result in an increase in drug usage. In the Netherlands, where cannabis has not, as is often stated, been legalized or even decriminalized, but where possession of small quantities of cannabis is ignored by the police and where sale of cannabis in 'coffee shops' is tolerated by the authorities, the rates of highly addictive drug usage have stabilized at a low level in comparison to most other European countries. Rates of cannabis usage have also stabilized and indeed are now reducing somewhat.

All this presupposes effective education. As in the case of alcohol education, the studies of the effectiveness of drugs education are not encouraging. But there are now indications that drug usage can be reduced if education is directed at the whole community and not just at schoolchildren. Those American programmes, described in the Royal College of Psychiatrists Report, that include interactive methods (giving the young the opportunity to debate as well as to listen), as well as a parents' component, that are long-term over the whole school career, that are family-focused, that are combined with media campaigns and policy changes, that include community programmes to strengthen norms against drug use, and that are sensitive to the age of the child as well as culture-sensitive, do have encouraging effects. One study of 14-year-olds along these lines found 44% fewer drug users and 66% fewer users of multiple drugs in an intervention group compared to an untreated control group six years later. Such programmes are, it must be said, not available in the UK or indeed in most parts of the United States, but the fact that programmes with demonstrable effectiveness do exist must give encouragement to those who wish we could find more powerful ways to deter the young from playing with fire that may scar them for life for the sake of short-term enjoyment.

The great majority of young people in their teens choose not to use drugs or only to use them in modest amounts that stand very little chance of harming them. It is surely the responsibility of the adult world to try to make sure that those at risk of entering the dangerous world of heavy drug usage are well informed before they make this choice. And for those who have become drug-dependent, we need better services to meet their needs.

Chapter 8

Eating well and feeling good

8.1 Introduction

There are two prevalent myths about the teens and their attitudes to food, appetite, and appearance. One is that they are all overweight because they are so inert and watch television or videos the whole time; the other that they are all on the verge of anorexia. Because this is a time of rapid growth, the calorie needs of those in their teens are indeed greater than at other times of life. Teenagers do eat more food. Most have an appetite that is somewhere between healthy and ravenous. Further, as we shall see, many teenagers, especially girls, are distressed about their appearance and are trying to do something about it. They are either embarking on a diet, actually dieting, or have just given up on a diet. But in fact about four in every five of them are a perfectly healthy weight, neither over- nor underweight and, contrary to media reports, most are in no danger either of anorexia or obesity.

So many of the myths around food and the teens are quite misleading. All the same, by the time young people reach their early teens an increasing number, perhaps one in five compared to one in ten only 20 years ago, do weigh more, some far more than they should. They are, quite reasonably, unhappy about it. They don't like the look of their bodies and their weight is indeed unhealthy. Further, if young people arrive at their early teens overweight their chances of reaching their twenties in better shape are small.

In this chapter, I shall concentrate on overweight, dieting, and anorexia, but the preoccupation of young people with appearance, aided by the media, extends well beyond the issue of size. Increasingly, young people in their teens are becoming dissatisfied with other aspects of their appearance and are beginning to wonder whether they can be remoulded by cosmetic surgery. This trend is already apparent in the United States. According to Alissa Quart, in a survey carried out by *Seventeen* magazine in October 2000, not only had 25% of readers considered liposuction, tummy tucks, or breast augmentation, but 12% had considered a 'nose job'. A number of UK teenagers have already started to press plastic surgeons to operate on them.

8.2 **The overweight teens**

Why does overweight and its extreme form, obesity, occur? There are, as is well known, only two reasons for people being overweight, whatever age they might be. They either eat too much or take too little exercise. The fact that one in five young people in their teens are overweight might make us think that eating too much and taking too little exercise is only a problem for a relatively small minority. But this would be misleading. In fact, the average weight of the whole population of children and young people is greater than it was 20 years ago. This means it is virtually inevitable that there are now more seriously overweight young people than there used to be. Just as, if the average income of the whole population increases it is highly likely there will be more millionaires and if the average amount of alcohol we drink goes up there will be more alcoholics, so if the average weight of the population goes up we must expect there to be more obese or seriously overweight people. So, if we want to have fewer seriously overweight young people, apart, of course, from trying to help those who are affected in this way in the extremely difficult task of reducing their weight, we have to think what measures might result in the average weight of the whole population coming down.

Who should take responsibility for reducing the average weight of children and young people? The most obvious answer to this question is that parents should take responsibility for diet and exercise as far as children are concerned, and young people themselves should take responsibility once the teen years are reached. It is not that easy.

Nell is a 15-year-old girl who went through puberty a little early and is fully sexually mature. She has reached her adult height of 5 feet 6 inches (167 cms), and is a little taller than her mother. She weighs 12 stone (76 kg). This gives her a 'body mass index' of 27, which makes her heavier than 98 out of 100 girls of her age. Nell, like most obese girls of her age has been overweight since early childhood. Indeed, when she was at infant school, her teacher suggested that her mother take her to the doctor for this problem, and her mother tried unsuccessfully to limit her food intake right through her childhood. Now she is a cheerful girl, who is popular at school, and has lots of girlfriends. She just loves food. She certainly looks plump. Unlike most of the girls in her class, perhaps partly because she is an unfashionable shape, she does not have a boyfriend. This does not particularly upset her. Like most of her girlfriends, she spends a lot of time listening to music, watching television and videos, and takes very little exercise. Every six months or so she goes on a diet and loses a few pounds, but then after about a fortnight of misery, goes to a party, eats more than she is supposed to on her diet and gives up on it. Her mother, with whom she gets on well, is mildly overweight, also goes on a diet from time to time and then gives up. She takes the view that it is up to Nell to decide what to do about her weight. About a year ago, the two of them made a big effort together to lose weight together, but it led to a lot of tension between them when Nell began to give up and they both decided this was not something they should try again.

Nell's overweight means that she is at increased risk of being obese throughout her adult life and of developing diabetes, arthritis, gall bladder disease, heart disease, and an early death. Indeed the risk of diabetes has gone up quite considerably in recent years, because of the increase in the numbers of seriously overweight children and adolescents. Even now, Nell's weight affects her quality of life, because she gets out of breath easily when she exercises. Although she is generally cheerful, her failure to lose weight by dieting does distress her. We do not know why precisely Nell is overweight when so many of her friends are not. Because 17 out of 20 pre-school children consume more sugar than the recommended maximum, it is highly likely Nell did too. Because sweets, biscuits and pastries, soft drinks, chocolate, crisps, savoury snacks account for 39% of the energy intake of British pre-school children, while vegetables, fruit and nuts account for only 5%, it is highly likely Nell's diet was very high in sugar and salt at that time. Nell has probably been eating more saturated fat than the recommended maximum since she went to school, since this is the case for nine out of ten British schoolchildren.

So Nell, like most young people of her age, has been on an unhealthy diet from her early childhood and throughout her school years. Also like most British and American young people (see Chapter 9), she exercises very little. Why should Nell be so overweight when most of her friends weigh distinctly less? It may be that she has been eating somewhat more and exercising somewhat less than they have. But it is also probable that the genes she has inherited from her parents have made her vulnerable to put on more weight than others in a world where most children and indeed most adults are eating unhealthily. So in order to understand Nell's problem, we have to look at the reasons for unhealthy eating more generally.

How the world in which parents and young people live makes healthy eating difficult. As the 2001 Food Commission Report makes clear, food advertising accounts for 7 out of 10 advertisements on children's weekday ITV and 5 out of 10 advertisements on Saturday morning children's programmes. About 19 out of 20 adverts are for foods high in fat and/or sugar and/or salt. Partly because of subsidies to sugar production, healthy foods are more expensive. There is a strong link between obesity and low income. Poor families cannot afford to eat healthily. Until recently, and there has certainly been a change in official

British government attitudes over recent years, most schools have taken little interest in the provision of healthy school meals or in the unhealthy content of lunch boxes brought to school. In some schools, soft drink/confectionary machines and tuck shops have been used to generate revenue for the school. The school curriculum has generally been thin on information on healthy eating.

The commercial pressure generated by the relative price of healthy and unhealthy food, as well as the highly targeted advertising of unhealthy food means that parents, like Nell's mother, have an uphill task to ensure their children eat well. Then, when their children reach the teen years and take responsibility for their own food intake to a greater degree, many of them, like Nell, are so overweight that they cannot realistically be expected to lose significant amounts of weight and, even if they do, maintain their weight at a healthy level. Most of them are eating unhealthily and are relatively powerless to do anything about it. So they go on diets and, as we shall see, dieting is a significant source of unhappiness.

8.3 Dieting and unhappy: the normal state of the female sex today

Most girls in their teens and quite a number of boys are worried about the amount they eat. They are not so concerned about their weight, much more about their appearance. Dieting is a major preoccupation for them. Their worries may be at their most intense in the teen years, but they begin earlier and, as far as many people are concerned, they continue throughout life.

Round about the age of nine or ten, at the beginning of puberty or just before it begins, children start to make the link between the amount they eat and the way they look; they realize they can take responsibility for their own food intake. In the UK, psychologists Hill and colleagues studied 170 girls aged 9 and 14 years at an independent school in Yorkshire. By 14 years, 70% of them had dieted at some time and 30% were currently dieting. The degree to which the girls dieted increased over the five years from 9 to 14 years, but quite a few of the children were already dieting at nine years old and many more were conscious of their weight. At both ages, the girls on diets had more dissatisfaction with their bodies and lower self-esteem than others. Although the girls who dieted were, on average, heavier than those who didn't, almost half the girls who were dieting were not overweight.

Girls in Sweden diet even earlier. A study there revealed that around one in five 7-year-olds said they had tried to lose weight by dieting, probably at the suggestion or insistence of their parents. Certainly by 10 or 11 years old, many children, especially if they are girls and especially if they are plumper than average, begin to diet independently of their parents' wishes. Because of the increase in the size of buttocks and breasts that occurs naturally during puberty, this means that those who enter puberty earlier are also those who start dieting earlier.

Dieting continues throughout adult life. At any one time, about half the adult female population is either embarking on a diet, is actually on a diet, or has just given up a course of dieting. Men diet about half as often, but still very frequently. Dieting behaviour is prevalent right through to old age. So dieting is not, as is sometimes suggested, exclusively a teenage preoccupation. It does not even begin in the teens let alone end there. It is currently a lifelong obsession.

Cheryl is now 25 years old. She shares a flat with another young woman a year or two older, and has a good social life. She doesn't have a regular boyfriend at the moment, but she has had two quite long relationships in the past, and is currently enjoying her freedom. Her job as a computer technician is interesting and not badly paid. In most ways she is fit and well and her weight is unremarkable. She weighs ten and a half stone, just a bit above average for her height of five feet, five inches. Yet it would be misleading to say that Cheryl is happy with her health. In particular, she is dissatisfied with her weight and appearance. She has not really been happy about this since she was 7 years old. In fact, since her birth, Cheryl's mother had worried about her tendency to put on weight and had tried, ineffectively, to limit the amount she ate. By the age of 7 years, Cheryl was fond of looking at the teen magazines her older sister, then 13 years of age, bought. She started looking at herself in the mirror and decided she was too fat. Her mother, who was then in her late thirties, was quite slim and much concerned about her own appearance, told her not to be silly, though she was secretly worried that Cheryl was indeed going to be unfashionably plump. Her father laughed at her and just told her not to be ridiculous.

When her breasts began to develop at around the age of 10 years, Cheryl found herself in a group of highly fashion conscious little girls. For the first time she began to try to control how much she ate. Since that time, indeed for the whole of the last 15 years, she has been engaged in a struggle to achieve a weight just a bit below what seems to be her natural weight. She has never properly enjoyed a hearty meal without feeling she was harming her appearance. This has not stopped her eating a vast quantity of fast food, especially in her early and mid-teens, though since her late teens she has been eating more healthily.

Cheryl began to smoke when she was 11 years old. Her older sister smoked at that time as did her mother and there were always free smokes around at home. She has tried to give up but always puts on weight when she does and can't lose weight sufficiently to satisfy herself when she is not smoking. Now she smokes 15 cigarettes a day. When she was 15 she tried a joint, but didn't take to it and hasn't tried them out again. She has never drunk much alcohol, and usually drinks mineral water when out with friends. At 18, she left school and did a one year computer course. Since then she has only had two jobs, the present one for over four years. Her diet and smoking habits have changed very little since she left school.

After last Christmas, using some of her bonus, Cheryl took out a year's subscription to join a health club. She went three times, but hasn't been back since, and it is now April. She finds exercise too boring.

Cheryl's story is typical of many. It is not that she is in any way clinically depressed. But she is constantly dissatisfied with her appearance and her self-esteem about her appearance is low. It would be misleading to say she is really unhealthy. She pants a bit going up two flights of stairs at work, and she tends to cough a little in the mornings. No more than that. Yet she is building up trouble for the future, not with respect to her weight, but because she smokes. She can see this for herself because her mother, now in her mid-fifties, has a smoker's cough with chronic bronchitis and, for the first time in her life, is getting seriously overweight.

It would be easy to say that Cheryl has brought all this on herself and, in an important sense, she has. No one forced her to eat unhealthily or to take up smoking. No one is stopping her from taking regular exercise and she has the resources to do this if she wants to. Yet it would also be true to say that pressures from the society in which she has lived, have made it very difficult for her to make better choices.

As Cheryl's story shows, unhealthy lifestyle habits begin well before the teens and sometimes last the whole of the rest of life. Though the teens are often blamed for them, they are not particularly teen problems. Cheryl began to smoke and eat unhealthily well before puberty. She took little exercise at that time too. These habits continued into her mid-twenties and it is likely they will continue into her old age.

In the view of experts on eating problems, Cheryl would be regarded as a 'normal' dieter. She is, of course, normal, in the sense that most young women of her age share her preoccupations about appearance and most have had similar, perhaps even more intense preoccupations about dieting in adolescence. But is it right that Cheryl should be regarded as 'normal' in this respect, when her appearance is a cause of such dissatisfaction? Is there not something amiss in a society that creates such a feeling of failure in so many of its women, both young and old? In particular, should she have gone through her teen years with such an unnecessary feeling of disappointment in her appearance?

Cheryl, like so many young women, went through the teens feeling powerless to achieve the bodily shape she was encouraged to believe she should have.

She felt 'landed', even in her early teens, with a body she did not want. And it was the adult world, the world making money out of publishing teen and women's magazines, promoting fashion consciousness in clothes manufacture and retailing, and selling diets of one sort or another that was responsible for her chronic dissatisfaction with herself and the way she looked.

8.4 Anorexia nervosa: girls who starve themselves

Fortunately, although dissatisfaction with appearance and dieting is the norm for teenage girls, only about one in a hundred starve themselves to a degree that seriously threatens their physical health and takes over their lives to the exclusion of everything else. Such girls spend all their waking hours preoccupied with food. They stop having their periods or, if the problem arises before periods have started, these are delayed or just do not occur. For about a third of girls with anorexia nervosa, the problem will continue well into adulthood and perhaps for the rest of their lives, making it difficult for them to have ordinary social and sexual relationships. They are unlikely to get married, and if they do and have children, the way they feed their children will be affected. About a third will recover from the problem completely after a few months or a year or two. The lives of the remainder will be affected, often for years, but they will be able to lead a pretty normal life. They may be able to look back at the way they starved themselves in adolescence and joke about it. But for the seriously affected, anorexia nervosa is no joke. About one in ten eventually commit suicide or die from starvation.

Anorexia is an illness partly arising out of the social pressures to diet, with young people, especially young girls powerless to resist the media hype to slim. But it is also a method young girls use to win control from their parents when they can see no other way of escaping powerlessness within the family. Anorexia has also been seen as a way of fighting against the changes that sexual maturity brings, avoiding the challenge of womanhood by keeping the body childlike. All three of these explanations involve young people desperately trying to gain control in situations in which they feel powerless. It is when these three forms of powerlessness are combined and, in addition, a girl is vulnerable because of the genes she has inherited, that the illness, and it is an illness, occurs.

Louise is a 15-year-old girl who had always seen herself as a little overweight, started to diet more obsessionally than her friends three years ago. After they had read about it in a magazine, they all started a new diet together, but whereas the others gave up after a few days or at most a few weeks, Louise did not seem to know when to stop. Now she is skeletal in appearance, in danger of dying from malnutrition, and on the verge of a compulsory admission to hospital. She had

not started her periods when the illness began and she has in fact never menstru-
ated. No one can understand how all this came about. Louise was apparently
a happy girl, perhaps a trifle over-serious and inhibited, but that was to be
expected because both her parents were rather solemn people with an intense
attitude to life. They were active in their local church and, despite the fact that
they were both busy and successful in their work (Louise's father is an accountant
in a London city firm, and her mother a deputy head teacher in a primary school)
were dedicated to service in the community.

There was nothing much unusual about the family. Louise attended a private
school, and got quite a lot of homework, which she completed without difficulty,
though she took a great deal more time over it than most girls in her class. But she
never protested. She was usually near the top in most subjects. Her parents had
both been academically successful at school, and expected their daughter to
achieve similarly, especially as her older brother had won a scholarship to
a Cambridge college, where he was to start the following October. Family life was
busy, and there wasn't much time for chat. The communication that did occur
usually revolved around who was going to be in first to feed the dog and take him
for a walk, what was going to be left for supper in the fridge (as the commitments
of the members of the family rarely allowed them to eat together), and which
church service they would attend next Sunday.

Now Louise has anorexia nervosa, life is very different. On the advice of
their family doctor, guided by a consultant child psychiatrist, the family members
always eat together in the evening. It is thought that Louise cannot be trusted
to eat adequately if she is left to her own devices. They have all had to give up
their other evening activities. During supper, all eyes are on Louise as she toys
with her food. Her parents have been told she is not to leave the table until she has
finished all on her plate. But this is not working. She sits there for hours. Her par-
ents have tried ignoring, cajoling, shouting, bribing, and threatening her, nothing
seems to work. From being the young mouse everyone took for granted, Louise has
become the most powerful member of the family. But she has had to pay with her
health.

Now Louise would never have developed anorexia if she had not embarked
on the diet recommended by the magazine. On the other hand, the diet was
clearly not the only factor involved. After all, her friends went on the same
diet but did not develop it. So there must have been other forces at work. In
girls like Louise, it usually turns out that, although they have always been very
obedient children, indeed often unusually obedient, this has been at a cost.
They have been unable to express their real feelings about what they are expected to do. Often, though by no means always, this revolves around an underlying rebellious attitude to schoolwork and examinations. It is easy to blame

parents for putting undue academic pressure on their children, but they too may be in a powerless position in a society that values academic achievement and success in examination to the degree it does.

Family therapists have pointed to the lack of communication, especially lack of emotional communication between family members. These differences may exist, but their importance as a cause of the problem has been exaggerated. Many, probably most communication problems arise because of the tension produced by the anorexia and not the other way round.

All the same, it is true that, in some families with a girl suffering from anorexia, it is difficult for parents to express their feelings to each other. So, not surprisingly, it is hard for their children to communicate how they feel to them. Some parents of self-starving adolescents do not credit their children with feelings of their own. They speak for them. In interviews when the whole family is present, typically the interview goes like this: 'How do you manage in PE, if you are so worried other girls might see how thin you are?' a therapist might ask of a teenage girl. 'Oh, we don't worry about that, do we? Other children are too busy changing to notice us,' the mother might reply on behalf of her 15-year-old daughter, thus subtly, or perhaps not so subtly, removing her sense of personal identity from her. So self-starvation in a young girl with anorexia is often seen by therapists as a means of gaining power in situations where she feels unable to assert her independence as an individual with her own needs in any other way.

Here are some extracts from accounts given by people with anorexia nervosa to psychiatrist Arthur Crisp about the way they saw their illness arising:

> 'I was surrounded by a united family who loved me ... yet at the same time I sensed a disapproval of all the feelings that were stirring within me ... then a powerful force inside me, stronger than anything I've ever known before or since, dictated that I must embark on a course of self-starvation ... I was intoxicated by a sense of power ...'.

> 'During the last five years my life has been one long struggle to escape the strong but subtle domination of my mother .... I suppose that it was the need to prove my own identity that made me challenge my mother's authority ... anorexia is very much a family problem .... My mother has a wonderful skill of being polite .... She is marvellous at covering uncomfortable feelings ... Her niceness has been noted with wonder by neighbours ... and it is not surprising that I was made to feel guilty for challenging her ... I have tried hard to speak and act with Mum as a friend and equal but the relationship rarely lasts more than a week and then I return to my old state of despair and depression ...'.

> 'Going back to why I stopped eating. I have never pinpointed why I did it ... After talking with the psychiatrist it was a type of rebellion against my parents for sending me to boarding school.'

'During my teens I was aware of the distinct but certain knowledge that my father strongly disapproved of discos, parties and boyfriends; the usual paraphernalia of adolescence. Unconsciously therefore I buried myself in an ever growing mound of schoolwork ... became withdrawn and depressed. This decline accelerated rapidly one school holiday while my father was in hospital. My mother was swamped by the demands of home and office, and I was left alone and I soon enmeshed myself in a cast iron discipline of schoolwork and dieting. I lost weight rapidly ...'.

But there must be more than media pressures to diet and communication problems within families to explain anorexia. Otherwise, about half the girls in single-sex schools would suffer from it and, although there is certainly concern about rising rates of anorexia, the numbers of girls who do actually develop the full-blown illness is tiny. Clearly the girls who do develop anorexia are vulnerable in some other way and, not surprisingly, genes and genetic influence complete the picture.

Studies of identical and non-identical twins with anorexia suggest those who get the disorder differ from the rest by being genetically vulnerable. In a society with less pressure and role conflict, these genetically vulnerable girls would not develop anorexia. On the other hand, in a society where more girls experienced such conflicts as well as pressure to diet, even those with lesser genetic vulnerability would develop the disorder.

One of the ways in which girls show their genetic vulnerability is in their personalities. Those who starve themselves in this way are often highly conscientious and perfectionist. From an early age they have liked order in their lives. They tend to timetable themselves rigidly and like everyone else to be punctual as well. They love to be helping other people and often have ambitions to spend their lives in some form of service. They may want to become doctors, nurses, or work in paramedical occupations. Alternatively, they like the idea of being flight attendants or working in the catering trades, serving other people with food they cannot stomach themselves. Their ability to control their weight is often a matter of pride and part of a desire to control all aspects of their lives. They hate the idea of their feelings getting out of control. This need for control, especially over food, has often been present since earlier childhood; indeed many have had feeding difficulties when they were toddlers.

8.5 Anorexia: intoxication with power

Girls with anorexia often say, as did the young woman quoted earlier, that the control they have achieved over their bodies by self-starvation gives them an incredible feeling of liberation, of at last achieving a sense they can control their own destinies. The problem is that the sense of release is only achieved at the cost of sacrificing their health, as well as their good relationships with family and friends. If their lives are in danger, though they try to avoid it, they just have to come for psychiatric treatment. Paradoxically, the psychiatrist, in order to save life, is then forced to take away their liberty and ensure they do eat. As was the case with Louise, parents are told they have to take firm control and ensure their children do eat. However, once the girl's life is out of danger, this process can be reversed. All the therapeutic effort is put into understanding the girl's need for control and to help her find for herself other ways of achieving the power she feels she has lost. Such psychotherapy is usually successful in bringing about at least partial improvement.

8.6 **Bulimia: bingeing and losing control**

Although it nearly always occurs for the first time in the late teens and early twenties, bulimia, self-induced vomiting after bingeing, has much in common with anorexia. About one in three girls and young women with bulimia have had anorexia in the past. Most are not chronically overweight, though they may well have 'weight swings'. Most improve as they move into and through their twenties, but a minority are chronically affected. As with anorexia, young people with bulimia often have a deep sense of failure and powerlessness, not only over their body shape, but in other areas of their lives.

Seeing dieting, anorexia, and bulimia as reflecting different ways of responding to lack of power gives meaning to these forms of behaviour and makes them understandable not just for the young person who is affected but also for the whole adolescent age group, disempowered as it is in so many different ways.

There are many ways in which those who make public policy as well as those who are involved in the media could help to reduce the likelihood of young people developing both overweight and anorexia.

As far as overweight and obesity are concerned, they could:

- Recognize that overweight problems begin in early childhood and are much, more difficult to deal with in later life. Consequently they could put more resources into parent education regarding diet and physical activity in the early years.
- Incorporate a much more substantial component of nutrition into the physical education curriculum in schools in order to empower the young to monitor their own intake (food) and energy output (exercise).
- They could ensure the same messages are delivered (reduction of TV, video viewing, and playing of computer games; decreasing consumption of high fat foods; increasing fruit and vegetable intake; and increasing vigorous

physical exercise) into other parts of the school curriculum. Steven Gortmaker and his colleagues in the United States showed they could reduce the amount of obesity in 12–14-year-old girls by introducing lessons along these lines into the language arts, maths, science, and social studies as well as the physical education curriculum.

◆ Making healthier food a reality in schools by providing it at breaks, lunch times, and breakfast clubs and making unhealthy foods unavailable. After all, schools don't provide cigarette machines in schools just because many students would find it convenient for them to do so.

◆ Ban television advertising of food and drink at least during television programmes initially for pre-school and then for pre-teen children.

◆ Greatly increasing the number and attractiveness of leisure facilities in the community to which the young have access. This is discussed further in Chapter 10.

When it comes to the prevention of anorexia, it seems important to recognize that western industrial society puts across very clear messages about the overwhelming importance of a slim appearance for success. The way girls, young women, and indeed older women look defines their identity. Warmth of personality, a caring attitude to other people, and capacity for enjoyment of the good things of life all tend to be subordinated to the need to look good. Arthur Crisp, the authority on anorexia mentioned earlier, has commented on a study carried out by Anne Becker and her colleagues of the way disordered patterns of eating in Fijian secondary schoolchildren appeared for the first time after the introduction of television to their islands in the 1990s. He refers to this effect of western society on those who, as a result of the phenomenon of globalization, have become exposed to it as 'a tale of corruption'. It is difficult to see it in any other way. Those who have lived in the West have been corrupted in a similar manner for several decades.

All this may sound exaggerated. After all, the media and the fashion industry that promote appearance, narrowly defined, as the ultimate criterion of female success are by-products of the commercial world and freedom of expression. Business may create consumer demand, but ultimately it is consumers who decide whether they want the product business offers. What can be done to try to ensure that consumers in the West ultimately change their values so that there is less universal dissatisfaction and disappointment among girls and young women over their appearance, together with fewer cases of anorexia? Those who make policy could:

◆ Make Personal, Social and Health Education (PSHE) in schools part of the National Curriculum rather than an optional extra. Part of the curriculum in this subject could involve to a greater degree than at present the way in which taste in fashion is manipulated for commercial reasons.

◆ Some of the content of the curriculum in other subjects such as English and History could be used to provide opportunities for discussion of the place of appearance in the value systems of characters in novels and plays, as well as those living in historical times.

◆ Stresses in school likely to impinge especially on those vulnerable to anorexia could be reduced. The British secondary school student is currently subject to more public examinations than are students in any other country. The significance of examination results for University entry requirements could be reduced. As things stand at present, it is the most able and academically successful students who have to take most tests. Surely it is those students who are having most difficulty whose progress needs to be most closely monitored, but preferably not by examinations.

◆ More time could be given in the school curriculum to subjects such as drama, art, and music that allow self-expression, thus reducing the inner tensions often present in depression and anorexia.

In the meantime, parents and young people themselves have to avoid these twin hazards of obesity and anorexia in present day society rather than in one they might wish to see. There is much they can do. Weight control in the early years, when parents are in a good position to supervise the amount their children eat, is certainly not impossible or a waste of time. By the teen years, those young people who are already overweight are going to have their work cut out to make an impact. If they are obese the effort will be worthwhile. Those who are a reasonable weight do not, by any means, face an impossible task to avoid becoming overweight. It is important for their later health that they make the effort to do so.

How can parents help? They can:

◆ Build up the confidence of their children by showing them they approve of how they look. If their teenage girls are overweight they can avoid pointing this out. Instead, whatever their size and shape, they can help them to dress so as to look good and then admire rather than bemoan their appearance.

◆ Try to take a similar attitude to their own appearance. If parents are constantly expressing dissatisfaction with their own appearance, it is not surprising their teenage children do the same.

◆ They can encourage taking exercise. Weight gain only occurs if energy output (exercise) is greater than energy input (food). Though both are helpful, taking exercise can be an easier way to lose weight than dieting.

Buying a tennis racket or a subscription to a health club can be a better investment than purchasing yet another book on dieting.

- They can keep the fridge and deep freeze free of calorie rich foods and full of vegetables and fresh fruit. They can keep crisps, biscuits, sweets, and chocolates out of the cupboards.

- If their children are way over the top as far as weight is concerned, they can encourage them to consult the family doctor. Obesity clinics do not have a great record of success, but there is evidence from the United States that supervised treatment involving a weight watchers approach with encouragement to exercise can have an effect in some young people.

- Stop worrying and let their children find contentment whatever their size or shape.

When it comes to anorexia it must be admitted that sometimes children are so vulnerable, perhaps because of their genetic makeup and personality, there is no way that parents can take action to prevent them from suffering from it. There is, in fact, no proven effective means of prevention, even for less vulnerable children. All the same, it seems sensible for parents to try to avoid those situations known to be linked to the illness. They can do this by:

- Taking steps to avoid being obsessed with their own appearance and level of thinness. There is a close link between the dissatisfaction with appearance felt by parents and their teenage children, so the more relaxed parents can be about their own attitudes to dieting and exercise, and the way they themselves look, the less likely it will be their children will fall into this trap.

- Trying to show they like the way their teenage child looks thus building up confidence about appearance.

- Keeping communication lines open by really listening to what their teenage children say, thus seeing the world from their perspective.

- Avoiding imposing their own ideas about homework, examinations, academic success, and university entry.

- Encouraging the idea of three or four family meals a week. Even family meals taken around a TV set are better than meals eaten in isolation.

- Noticing possible first signs of anorexia. These include refusing to sit down to eat meals with the rest of the family, being quite excessively picky and calorie conscious, and taking what seem to be ridiculous amounts of exercise in an obsessional way. Remember though that dieting is virtually universal among young people (and, as we have seen, not only young people), while true anorexia is quite unusual. If a young person of teen age shows more than one of these signs of anorexia, it is sensible to encourage them to consult a doctor or at least talk about the situation with someone they trust. The earlier anorexia is spotted and help obtained, the easier it is to treat successfully.

◆ If a young person does not seem to be able to stop losing weight, or her periods stop, and she refuses to go to see a doctor, parents should consult the doctor themselves to discuss the situation. It may even be advisable for some sort of compulsion to be used. This is very definitely a last resort, but it is important to remember that anorexia can be a fatal condition. There are times when parents have to step in and prevent such a tragedy.

Fortunately, most girls and young women, as we saw right at the start of this chapter, manage to steer a course between obesity and anorexia despite the pressures from society that encourage unhealthy eating of one sort or another. All the same, the adult world should surely try to make it easier than it is now for those vulnerable young people who are at risk of either of these problems to avoid them successfully.

Chapter 9

Schools: the solution or the problem?

Education is empowering. Without educational success young people are condemned to low paid jobs, a much higher likelihood of unemployment and inability to appreciate many of the good things of life. But inevitably, from the perspective of those in their teens, making schooling compulsory risks being seen as disempowering. One can understand how they feel. Highly competent young people have the freedom to decide how they will spend their weekdays taken away from them until the age of 16 years. Even after that, the job market and benefits system, with no minimum wage protection and no allowance to benefit under 18 years, are arranged in such a way that most have little choice but to continue in some sort of educational setting however boring or unrewarding they may find it.

From 1972, when the school leaving age was raised to its present level of 16 years, it has been the law that children up to this age just have to go to school. There are legal penalties if they don't. As I write, a mother of five has been sent to prison for 60 days because two of her teenage children have been persistently absent from school.

The idea that all children should *have* to go to school is relatively recent. As W B Stephens makes clear in his historical account of education in Britain, only 200 years ago, at the beginning of the nineteenth century, less than one in fifteen of children in Britain attended school. But by 1860 most children under the age of 11 years, even those in the working class, were in school. In 1870, the first Act making school compulsory was passed. Between 1870 and 1902, elementary education became both free and compulsory up to the age of 11 years. Indeed, by 1914 about three in five 14-year-old children were in school and, in 1918, school was made compulsory up to this age. At the end of the Second World War, through the 1944 Education Act, school was made compulsory up to the age of 15 years, and in 1972, the school leaving age was raised to 16 years.

Incidentally, no one has ever asked the young what they think about schooling being compulsory. As with all major issues concerning educational policy, decisions affecting the lives of children and young people have been taken largely by local and national politicians without, at least until the 1960s when parents' organizations promoting comprehensive education were established, involving parents let alone children and young people themselves. Discussions in parliament about such major educational issues as the importance of a technical education for later employability, the fairness of the 11+ examination, and the structure and content of examinations have all taken place with little attempt to find out what children and young people themselves would like. Instead, the argument has been dominated by politicians, the unions, and industry with the later addition of an initially weak and then much stronger parental voice. Later in this chapter, I shall quote views of young people about school which suggest that, though many might accept the need for compulsory attendance, they would prefer quite a different form of schooling.

9.1 **Teenagers for whom school is just made**

Jane is now in her early twenties. She was enthusiastic about school from the time she first attended at the age of five years. She made friends easily and was good at all the school subjects. Never top of the class, she nevertheless was a bright student all the way through. She got good results in the public examinations she took and is now a medical student at a London medical school. In her early years of secondary school, she was mildly disruptive because she found some of the lessons boring, having already covered some of the ground in her primary school. This problem was overcome after discussion between her teachers, her parents, and Jane herself. She was given some extra work that she found quite difficult, and this seemed to solve the problem. Otherwise she never really seemed to find school anything other than a pleasurable experience. School seemed to have been made for Jane.

9.2 **Teenagers who do not fit the school system**

Nick, now in his early twenties too, never liked school. He just failed to fit into the routine. He was often in serious trouble at his primary school for poor work when it was thought he could do better. He was the butt of sarcasm from teachers because he was silent when asked a question in class, though he was known to be talkative and popular with his friends. Although his art work was good, he was slow to read and could never do more than rudimentary work in maths. He didn't just dislike his secondary school; he hated it. Apart from the pleasure of seeing his friends, it seemed to have nothing to offer him. The art teaching failed to inspire him and this was the only subject that interested him. He played truant from the age of 13 whenever he thought he could get away with it. His parents knew about his truancy, but could not persuade him to attend more regularly. Their visits to talk to his teachers were unpleasant experiences for the teachers, who were made to feel failures, as well as for them. They got the impression that the school thought Nick's attendance was their fault. When the school authorities caught up with him, he attended just enough to get them off his back. He left school at the first opportunity and got a job filling shelves at the local supermarket. A year later, with some help from his parents, he upgraded the home computer and began to experiment with some of the more sophisticated design software he saved up to buy from his small earnings. He found that he could master this quite easily. He went to a computer design course for a year that he attended very regularly and did well. By the age of twenty he had got himself a reasonably paid job and had put his school years behind him.

9.3 **What do the young think of school now?**

Whose experience is the more typical, and what do those whose lives have been most affected by the introduction of compulsory schooling think about what has been done for their benefit? The survey evidence suggests that being forced to go to school has, in general, not gone down well with most young people in their mid-teens. We have little systematic information about how children in past times have regarded school, though what we do have in the way of autobiographical recollections is not complimentary. 'Fortunately for the size of the classes,' wrote Robert Roberts, for example, of the schooling he received in his teens in the early 1900s, 'anything up to a quarter of the pupils would stay away.' Laurie Lee describes his village schooling in the 1920s up to the age of 14 years, when he was at last able to leave. 'The narrow school was just a conveyor belt along which the short years drew us ...'. The last day of school was a 'lucky, lucky point of time; our eyes were on it always ... . There was no more to be done, no more to be learned. We began to look around the schoolroom with nostalgia and impatience ... . At last Miss Wardley was wringing our hands, tender and deferential. "Good-bye old chaps, and jolly good luck! Don't forget to come back and see me." She gave each one of us a coy, sad glance. She knew we never would.'

Since the raising of the school leaving age to 16 years we have more systematic information taken from surveys. In 1999, for example, Jacki Gordon and Gillian Grant report how around 1600 students aged between thirteen and a half and fourteen and a half in Glasgow secondary schools were asked on how they felt and many talked about school. Most expressed dissatisfaction. Of course, there were positive responses. Some enjoyed the lessons and obtained a feeling of achievement when they had mastered something they found difficult.

'In Chemistry, I finally worked out how you form all those molecules and junk like that!'

Others valued praise from teachers.

'In geography I found out that the teacher liked my work so I felt even happier and proud.'

Some linked the positive side of school to friendships rather than lessons.

'I've got Chemistry (I love it because I can talk to Craig, Paul and Tim through it), Computing (my friend Maggie sits next to me so I can talk to her) and French (Andy's there and he's hilarious). The best bit about school is the lunch break because I get to hang around with all my friends and we just have a laugh.'

But most had negative feelings. The most common response to the request to name 'three things that make me feel bad about myself' was doing badly at school. Complaints were especially to do with boredom.

'I am very bored. I wish I didn't have to go to school. School is very depressing although you learn stuff. The only good thing about it is playtime, dinnertime and home time and that's all.' 'I love weekends and live for weekends and holidays. I get through the week by thinking about the weekends.'

Some feel confined and trapped by school.

'I get bored with near enough all the subjects because I don't like the teachers. I feel as if I'm trapped because I have no choice in the matter about going to school. If I had my own way I wouldn't go near school.'

Others feel stressed by exams.

'Today I feel very stressed and under pressure. I have to learn so much in such a short time and I seem to be getting one test after another.'

Homework can mean that school stresses spill over into the home.

'You have a teacher moan at you all day long and when you go home your Mum will shout at you to do your homework. I think homework should be done in school so we don't get yelled at in the house.'

Teachers' attitudes are a reason for strong dissatisfaction.

'Just now I am sitting in English feeling very angry. I always seem to get picked on by this teacher, if everyone's forgot something or didn't do something she just picks on me even just for the simplest little thing. She screams at me in a horrible high pitched voice which just goes right through me.'

Teachers are not thought to deserve respect.

'I hate saying Sir. As if an old prick who has a degree needs to be called sir. Sometimes I contemplate confronting him, but I have to keep in with him or my life is a mess.'

And feelings can be intensely experienced.

> 'I wish I could just get away. I feel so depressed. I just can't cope with the work at school, suicide would be the easiest thing. I just hate my life.'

These are the views of mainly working class young people in Glasgow, but there is evidence they are shared throughout the UK. In a study of 30 000 secondary students carried out from Keele University in the mid-1990s, Michael Barber found as many as 10–15% truanted, nearly one in three said that others in their class disrupted lessons every day, and fully 60% agreed with a statement that they 'count the minutes' to the end of the lesson. It is not that these young people dislike school. Indeed nearly 90% say that they are happy at school; what is so worrying is that they find it such a disappointing experience. Such disappointment sets in after the first year at secondary school. As many parents and teachers will confirm, children generally arrive at their new schools at the age of 11 years all 'bright eyed and bushy tailed'. By the time they return after the end of their first year, many are cynical, disenchanted, and bored with their school experience. The Glasgow and Keele studies are further confirmed by work carried out by the National Foundation for Educational Research (NFER) quoted by Michael Barber that showed that among 14-year-olds:

- Over half say that most of the time they don't want to go to school;
- One in four thinks teachers are too easily satisfied;
- One in four admits to having played truant; and
- One in five denies being happy at school.

It is clear from reading the quotations from pupils in these studies that a large minority, perhaps over one in three, are largely turned off school and for a whole range of reasons. Lack of individualized teaching means that for many children, parts of the curriculum are too easy for some and too difficult for others. The first group are bored and the second frustrated. Many young people complain of poor teaching, with teachers unable to command respect because of their inability to keep order. A minority of teachers still use sarcasm and humiliating remarks to put down less able youngsters. In the early teens, physical bullying is still a common experience for boys, while being teased and harassed is part of the lives of many girls. For some children, Monday morning is a torment because of a physical fear they will be hurt. The frequent tests and examinations are found stressful, even by those students who are generally successful. Disruptive behaviour, usually by a minority of students, results in an unsettled atmosphere in the classroom in which it is hard for the majority to concentrate on learning.

The great majority of secondary school students, over 90% of young people, say they enjoy parts of the school day, especially sports and P.E., other favourite lessons, and seeing their friends. And for most of them, perhaps two in three, nearly every aspect of school, including the least popular formal subjects such as maths and the sciences, is worthwhile and enjoyable.

But can it be right that the adult world should force such a high proportion of young people between the ages of 11 and 16 years, as many as one in three, to undergo an experience every day during the week that so many of them find deeply unrewarding? Further, because of the lack of available employment in many parts of the country, even those in their later teens are more or less compelled to continue with their education, regardless of how satisfying or unsatisfying they find it.

In making school compulsory for all those in their teens up to the age of 16 years, and by ensuring that between 16 and 18 years it is almost impossible for young people to do anything else other than stay on in education, the state has taken on the responsibility for making the teen years a rewarding learning experience for all in their teen years. It is clear that the state has failed to fulfil this responsibility. Despite the large sums spent on our schools and the very substantial workforce of hard working teachers, many, and in some respects most young people of this age are unhappy about many of their school experiences. Why should this be and what can be done about it?

9.4 **The secondary school experience**

First, it is important to say that there is obviously a great deal that is right about schools; results are improving and many students do enjoy their time at school. But, as we have seen, from the perspective of the student, overall the news is not good. Why should this be? It is certainly not the fault of teachers, the vast majority of whom are hard working, dedicated to their task and to the welfare of students. One has to look more widely at different aspects of the educational system.

There are doubtless many reasons, and they will vary from area to area, from school to school, and from student to student, that why school is such an unrewarding experience for so many young people. Educational reform is high on the government agenda. There are many ways in which the educational system needs changing. In line with the theme of this book, the issue that I shall discuss here is the degree to which students can be, and sadly often are disempowered in school. I shall also suggest what, in many schools, though possibly in too few, is already being done to change the situation.

Largely secondary school students learn by listening to a teacher talking, asking questions if they don't understand, doing class work projects and home work that are marked individually and, periodically doing classroom and national tests and examinations to check progress and mark achievement. This approach is well suited to the well motivated, brighter students, but, even for them, there are various aspects of this typical experience that are disempowering. This need not be the case and, the school experience is increasingly being altered to ensure this is not so.

9.5 Means of empowering secondary school students

9.5.1 Providing feedback on teacher performance.

At the present time, if the teacher is boring, inaccurate or otherwise deficient, there is nothing the student can do about it apart from switching off. Equally, if not more importantly, the student has no formal opportunity to express satisfaction or gratitude to teachers no matter how superbly he or she is being taught. Generally, the student has no control or ability to monitor or comment on the quality of teaching. While the head teacher has responsibility for the quality of teaching in his or her school, and is responsible to the school governors in fulfilling this duty, neither the head nor the governors have anything approaching the knowledge of students to enable them to fulfil this task. Any knowledge that parents have about the quality of teaching is filtered through their children and is not first hand.

What is needed is a formal opportunity for students to provide feedback on their teachers on a regular basis. The UK government is now proposing that students' views are obtained as part of Ofsted inspections. However these only take place every three or four years. Much more frequent feedback is needed. If, in mid-school year, round about half way through the winter term, students were asked to complete anonymously a feedback form on their teachers and then to repeat the exercise at the end of the school year, this would enable teachers to respond to comments in time for the class making them to benefit. Of course, such information needs to be fed back confidentially and with sensitivity to teachers so that any risk of public humiliation is avoided.

By the time they reach secondary school age, or at least 13 or 14 years, students are capable of making such judgements in a thoughtful and constructive manner. They are able, for example, to recognize that some teachers are better at bringing on students with learning difficulties while others find it easier to teach brighter pupils. Such capacity might well not be present in many pupils of primary school age and it would certainly not exist in nursery school age children. This might seem obvious if it were not for the fact that Ofsted appears, at the time of writing, in August 2002, to be asking children as young as three years to make judgements about their teachers. Children of this age are going to be asked to choose between smiling and sad faces to describe their teachers. Empowerment is only meaningful if the person given extra powers is competent to use them; to do otherwise risks the whole concept of empowerment being given a bad name.

Experiments along these lines are currently taking place at the Samuel Whitbread School in Shefford, Bedfordshire. Here 35 students of all levels of ability have been trained to assess all newly qualified teachers and trainees. The ingredients of a good lesson, according to the students, seem very appropriate. Mutual respect between teachers and pupils, and good interaction between them figure prominently.

9.5.2 Selection of teaching staff

Involving them in selection of staff provides a further opportunity to empower secondary school students. In some UK secondary schools, students are already participating in this way. One secondary school head explained to Lynne Davies, who was carrying out a study of School Councils to be described in more detail below, 'The most exciting thing was the involvement in staff interviews. We used to have them show visitors round—but I thought I'd take it a bit further, and they had a certain perception of people ... so now from the moment the candidates arrive, pupils have responsibility. They take them round, talk to them. Then, when they have finished, pupils meet and decide the questions ... the brief I give them is, I want to know from you how well the person relates to young people, how you think you're going to get on, what sort of discipline and sanctions, how they are going to make lessons interesting ... pupils then come down to their governors' panel prior to the formal interviews for their views and feedback. Then, once the appointment is made, there is feedback to the pupils on who got the post, we explain the reasons why, and most of the time we have appointed the one they want.' In some Nordic countries, the process has gone further. For example, in Helsingborg, in south-west Sweden, schools are now, in a pilot scheme, putting students of 14 years and older onto interview panels for new teachers. The head teacher of one of the schools reported that he was satisfied with the results. A spokesman for the Swedish Teachers' Union said: 'It must be a support for the chosen teachers to know the students have had their say'. Experiments along these lines are just being undertaken in the UK. It is difficult to know why they should not be applied in all schools.

9.5.3 Choosing their own curriculum

If they decide to enter a course of study, adults choose what it is they want to learn. There is probably little sense in expecting primary school students to take an active part in deciding on their own curriculum. But by the time young people reach secondary school age, and certainly by the time they reach around the age of 13–14 years, they are quite capable of taking a major part in choice of subject. This already happens to a considerable degree when they enter courses for GCSEs. But subject choice is often made with little attention given to make sure that the student is as well informed as possible. Some schools do work very hard to inform them through parent's evenings and by arranging student to student contact. But how often do students have the opportunity to sit in on one or two lessons held for classes a year of two ahead of them in subjects they might choose so that they can have a real flavour of what they are letting themselves in for? To what degree do students have a real choice in which parts of a subject's curriculum they are to study? For example, how far do students choose their own set books in English Literature or their own period for historical study. Clearly there would be problems if students in a class made different choices in these matters, but a greater element of democratic participation might well be feasible.

9.5.4 Ensuring topics that empower are included in the National Curriculum

All knowledge is, to some degree empowering. Certainly without the basic skills of reading, writing, numeracy and, these days, information technology, students are lacking in the necessary competence to survive. Without literacy and numeracy skills, they cannot participate in the wider world, reading the newspaper, watching television, earning a reasonable living, filling in their tax forms. Without a grounding in the humanities, mathematics, and sciences, they cannot make decisions about the learning paths they wish to follow in the future and are denied what is everyone's right, namely access to the store of human knowledge. Subjects such as English, History, and the Physical and Biological Sciences are empowering because they enable the student in different ways to understand the world and the way it works. But there is a group of subjects currently excluded from the National Curriculum that are equally as empowering as basic skills and more so than most of the subjects currently compulsorily taught. These are grouped under the somewhat clumsy title of Personal, Health and Social Education (PSHE). Not only is PSHE a non-compulsory part of the curriculum, but there is a lack of facilities at a national level to train teachers to become skilled in teaching it.

There is ample evidence that children and, more especially young people aged 13–18 years do not think that school provides anything like an adequate preparation for adult life. The school curriculum prepares students for examinations, essential in the current state of the job market to find employment. But it pays little attention to what might be called life skills whether these are exercised in the home, in the work place, or in the wider world where relationships are made and broken. Many aspects of the existing curriculum also provide few opportunities for the exercise of creative imagination.

Of course, literacy and numeracy will always be essential requirements for anyone seeking employment. But increasingly employers are asking for people who can deliver more than examinations can test for. A good memory and the capacity to analyse a problem critically are still in demand. At least as important though is the ability to show flexibility, to think creatively and imaginatively, and to communicate effectively with other people. Effective communication requires more than the skill to transmit information. It requires emotional intelligence, allowing sensitive reactions to the emotions of those with whom one is dealing, and an awareness of one's own feelings and the way in which these may be affecting work relationships.

Increasingly it is seen to be part of a school's function to influence the lifestyle of its students in ways that act to improve health. Lifestyle is of paramount importance in influencing the health of individuals not only while they are children but in their later, adult life. Physical fitness, diet, smoking, alcohol and drug intake are the major factors affecting health and longevity. The teaching of PSHE is the main vehicle for influencing the lifestyles of the young.

How far does the existing secondary school curriculum provide for these needs? In many ways excellently in relation to the grounding in the humanities, mathematics, and the sciences; somewhat less well as far as making up for deficiencies in basic numeracy and literacy skills that have not been acquired in primary school; hardly at all in PSHE. Yet without the capacities that PSHE tries to promote many students will find themselves unable to capitalize on their knowledge store.

There is an assumption that parents will take main responsibility for the personal and social development of their children. Parents will indeed have a greater role here than in any other part of the school curriculum. But most parents looking at the PSHE 'non-statutory guidelines' will be daunted at the responsibility for covering such a wide range of topics. How many parents will feel happy to teach their children, quoting just a small fraction of the guidelines, 'to use a range of financial tools and services, including budgeting and saving, in managing personal money' or how to 'use the careers service', or 'about the options open to them post-16', or how to 'use assertiveness skills to resist unhelpful pressure', or about 'the link between eating patterns and self-image, including eating disorders', or how 'different forms of contraception work', or 'about the statutory and voluntary organizations that support relationships in crisis'?

9.5.5 **Empowerment through making the curriculum more relevant to the 'real world'**

Up to this point in time, the opportunities for a secondary school student to check up that what he is learning is going to be useful for him once he leaves school have been seriously limited. Another approach increasingly available to UK youngsters is 'work experience'. This usually involves 14–16-year-olds spending a fortnight in a work setting, such as an office, a clinic, or a bank. Most students use a computer during their work experience. There is preparation for the work, both for the students and for those in the workplace. Nearly all (98%) of placements are completed and they are popular with students. Those who go on such placements feel afterwards that they are more confident of working with adults and making friends at work, they have a better idea what it is like to go out to work, and they feel they have learned it is important to sort things out and solve problems on their own at work. One study of work experience placements found that over half of a group of students who went on them said that after their placement they felt more interested in doing well at school.

A fortnight is not a long time to prepare for the world at work. Surely what we need are more initiatives giving young people more prolonged periods of time at work, with the opportunity of earning some money at the same time. In a 2001 Green Paper, 'Building on Success', the British government now proposes to introduce more opportunities for young people of 14 years and older to spend more time in work placements, so that they can lay a foundation for entering an apprenticeship later on. This will mean that, from 14 to 16 years, they will be part-time in school and part-time at work. Although the teaching profession is suspicious of schemes that take young people out of school, there is every chance that young people will become more and not less engaged in school studies if they have the first hand opportunity to see how educational progress can help them find better and more interesting jobs.

9.5.6 **The use of teaching methods that engage and empower**

As all teachers know it is a major classroom challenge to engage children and young people actively in the learning process. How is this to be achieved? In a study of 4000 Scottish students carried out by Gray and his colleagues, the students were asked towards the end of their schooling what they found the most effective methods of learning and, in addition, what were the educational methods they most frequently encountered. Interactive teaching, giving students the opportunity to react to information, question it and debate it among themselves and with the teacher was thought to be the most effective teaching method. Listening to teachers lecturing was thought to be the least effective. Yet these students said that they had experienced far more lectures from teachers than lessons in which they had been encouraged to participate. The most common method of study was 'exercises, worked examples, prose and translations' (72%), followed by 'having notes dictated to you in class' (60%), and 'using dictated notes' (49%). Practical activity, class or group discussion, and creative activity, the teaching methods thought to be most effective, were all experienced by less than 20% of students.

Similarly, when Joan Ruddock and her colleagues in their study of school improvement asked groups of engaged and disengaged students how they felt schools could be improved, *both* groups put emphasis on what happens in the classroom. They said that 'school work needed to be made more interesting, that pupils should be given more opportunities to find things out for themselves, that classes needed to be smaller so the teacher will be able to get round better and help more people, that there was more active learning with more group work, and that teachers needed to learn to listen to pupils and explain things more'.

Teaching using interactive methods is more demanding and exhausting but also a great deal more interesting for teachers. Good lecturing involves meticulous preparation of material, but once that material is prepared, the only task that remains is to communicate it. In interactive teaching, the teachers role is to help students to process information actively by questioning and discussion. This virtually always results in teachers realizing that their information is more incomplete than they had realized. Students learn more about the fallibility of existing knowledge and are better able to express what is known in a particular subject area.

9.5.7 **Empowering by teaching others**

There are currently numerous initiatives involving the use of adult mentors drawn from the world of work or from the university student population to provide support for students, especially those finding their school experience difficult. But secondary school students can play this role themselves and indeed, as many teachers have discovered, be more actively engaged in learning by teaching. It is a common observation that the best way to make sure one has understood something is to try explaining it to somebody else. A class of 24 students with one teacher can, by dividing the class into 12 groups of two each, turn into a class of 12 students and 13 teachers. Some students naturally have the capacity to teach, many do not. Like most people, they have to be taught how to teach. The way children are taught how to teach will vary with their age and stage of development. But it has been well shown that 'reciprocal teaching' can be taught. A number of American studies have shown how teachers can indeed help students to use different teaching strategies and then to 'fade' themselves away from the teaching process, so that students can teach independently. Even in primary age children, small group teaching of students by students can result in really substantial improvement in reading comprehension scores and across other parts of the curriculum.

Successful teaching by students can occur across the age span. Again, Jackie Dearden has described how 15-year-olds from an inner city comprehensive school worked with 10- and 11-year-olds from one of its feeder primary schools. After a series of training sessions, the older students met and taught the younger ones once a fortnight over a period of two terms. Both the primary and secondary school pupils found the sessions worthwhile and academic gains were made. Overwhelmingly, the mentors felt that the experience had helped them accept responsibility and made them feel more responsible about themselves. The younger ones felt more positive about themselves and, in particular, more confident about going on to the next school. One said of her mentor, 'He has helped me to learn how to read and learn new words I haven't used before', and another, 'I'm starting to get clever'! Teachers involved in the scheme also generally felt positive.

9.5.8 Reducing disempowerment by limiting testing and examinations

Examinations are deemed necessary to ensure that the young have reached particular levels of attainment. The national examination system means that there is uniformity throughout the country, and that performance is nationally comparable. Requirements for university entrance necessarily involve examination results. Employers need examination results to gauge the ability of prospective employees. Tests or examinations provide the student with evidence of success.

All these reasons for examinations have some, though only some force. But it is also true that the examination culture removes power from students. Criteria for success and failure are set from outside in a process over which the student has no control. Examinations are also inimical to learning. Learning that is worth anything is carried throughout life, yet much of what is learned for examinations is forgotten once they have been taken. Learning takes place best when anxiety is at a moderate level, neither absent nor too intense; examinations produce almost intolerable stress in a significant number of students. Signs of over-examination are usually not difficult to spot. They include headaches, unwillingness to go to school, poor sleep, and inability to concentrate.

Learning is intended to bring about greater self-esteem in students; examinations create a sense of failure and reduce self-worth in the many students who, in their own eyes, do not do well or, any rate, not well enough.

In recent years the numbers of examinations has increased in all countries. Students in England take more than in any other European or north American country. They have to take national tests at 11 and 14 years. At 15 or 16 years they take GCSEs. In the year 2000, the so-called AS examination was introduced between GCSEs and 'A' levels. This means that students are either preparing or taking national or public examinations every year from the age of 14 years until they leave school or further education. The AS examination has further disturbed the balance between the need for examinations and the creation of a good learning environment. At the time of writing (July, 2003), there are welcome indications that there might be a radical reduction in the number of examinations taken. An influential committee has recommended a move to a Baccalaureat type of single examination or Diploma, assessing basic skills, specialist subjects, and the student's performance on a wider range of criteria, including engagement in sport and voluntary work outside school. Such a system is being pioneered in Wales with some success.

9.5.9 Empowerment by involving students in school organization

Over 95% of secondary school students obediently turn up for school each morning in term time but, as we have seen, this should not fool us into thinking that they all have a rewarding experience there. I noted earlier how at least a third are bored and frustrated a good deal of the time they are in school. Interactive, more engaging methods of teaching and giving them greater influence over setting their own curriculum would reduce disaffection, but we also need to look at ways to empower students more generally in the organization of their schools.

In the Report of the Advisory Group on Education for Citizenship and the Teaching of Democracy in Schools chaired by Bernard Crick and published in the year 1998, it is recommended that citizenship teaching should be an entitlement of all pupils. The Report speaks most positively of citizenship as involvement in public affairs, in the need to encourage social and moral responsibility, community involvement, and political literacy. It also warmly describes examples of school councils that have a clearly beneficial effect on the ethos of the school. However, the recommendations it makes are seriously disappointing in the degree to which they refer to students participating in the way their schools are run. Instead, emphasis is put on the academic understanding of democratic principles. There is no recommendation that all schools should have a Student or Pupil Council. In general, democratic principles are surely better learned by participation in an institution showing many features of democracy rather than by formal lectures or even by discussion of political or social issues. The subject of citizenship has now been incorporated into the National Curriculum, so that students will be introduced to academic knowledge in the field of what used to be called 'civics'. While this is to be welcomed, it is no substitute for giving students a taste of democracy in action through participation in school councils.

Involving students in the running of schools is bound to raise anxiety about taking responsibility from teachers, lowering educational standards, giving students the right to wander in and out of school or in and out of lessons as they wish, allowing unruly elements to gain control of the running of schools, exclusion of parents from involvement in school matters, and a whole set of other undesirable outcomes. But it is not necessary or desirable to think of students deciding what is taught, or doing all the teaching. It is obvious that, because of their inexperience, this would not be good for education, and indeed it is not what they would want. Nor does it mean that they should be the sole or even the main decision makers in how schools are run, what is taught and who does it. Being part of a democratic society means, among other things, that we all have to accept the will of the majority in many parts of our lives. Lawyers run their own chambers or firms of solicitors but work within a democratically agreed legal system. Civil servants work within structures agreed by national and local governments. But the more control civil servants have over their working conditions within the agreed structures the happier they are and, incidentally, evidence shows, the longer they live.

At least as importantly, involving students in the running of schools and consulting with them about the way the school functions does not mean that the aims and purposes, or what might be called the mission of schools should be set by students alone. In the democratic, liberal capitalist society in which we live, the mission of businesses, whatever their nature, is the making of profit for shareholders. The mission of central or local government departments is not set by those who work in them, but by ministers or elected members of local authorities. Employees do not decide on the aims and purposes of these organizations, though they work better and more efficiently if they are given a say in their running and some role in decision-making. The mission of schools is set by the government of the day and the elected members of the local authorities responsible for them, not by the students who attend them. If the voting age were lowered, as I suggest it should be in Chapter 11, then students would have a slightly greater input into deciding on the aims and purposes of schools, but no more than, for example, the employees in arms factories into the decision how much the country should spend on defence.

Schools, like factories, businesses, local government, and all other places of work, operate within a legal framework. In fact, giving students more say does not require any radical change in the legal framework of schools, though certainly some reforms will be necessary if meaningful change is to occur. Some change to the governance of schools is desirable. But most of what needs to change involves moving attitudes of teachers, parents, and students towards a greater sense of partnership resulting in less of an 'us and them' approach, more trust between these three stakeholders in education, and more interactive teaching methods.

At the beginning of the twenty-first century, there are finally signs that this is beginning to occur on more than a sporadic scale. As we have seen, Ofsted inspectors are now encouraged to obtain the views of students as part of the regular school inspection process. This is a wise move, for there are many aspects of school life in which students are most likely to know what is going on. In 1997, a 15-year-old girl, Sarah Briggs, wrote to her local newspaper complaining about slipping standards at her school. She wrote that she was worried for her exam prospects because teachers at her comprehensive in Mansfield, Nottinghamshire, were constantly taking time off. She argued that her school had not done enough to remedy defects identified by an official inspection, and that precious funds had been wasted on a visit by the Queen. 'Supply teachers are often late turning up for lessons because they don't know where they are supposed to be', she claimed. 'All this wastes time. Most of us don't feel prepared for our GCSE exam next year'. The school's response was to charge her with bringing the school into disrepute. The school wrote that she had been guilty of 'behaviour which brings the school into disrepute and could affect future pupil numbers'. She was ordered to write a formal letter of apology to the head teacher and staff for 'seriously disrespectful conduct'—or face expulsion. But she remained adamant. She stood by her comments and refused to apologize, insisting she had simply said what she thought was right. 'I won't say sorry just to get myself back in. I'd be lying to myself. Even if teachers disagree with what I've said there is no need for them to go this far'. Eventually Sarah got back to school, her expulsion overturned by the governors. But it would surely have been better for the educational standards in her school if she had had earlier access to Ofsted inspectors to make her case.

9.5.10 Student involvement in the prevention of bullying in schools

One of the most striking ways in which involvement of children and young people has been shown to make a difference is in cutting down on the bullying that goes on in schools. About one in eight young people report that they have been severely bullied in secondary school, and nearly half have been subject to less severe bullying. For a high proportion of young people of this age, going to school is a nightmare. They spend Sunday evening worrying about what they are going to meet the next day. While in school, their concentration is affected by fear of what will be done to them in the mid-morning break or in the dinner hour. The adult world has made school compulsory. There is no escape. At least an adult who is bullied in the workplace has the option to leave. Children in secondary school cannot choose to do that. One must seriously question the morality of a system that forces children into situations in which they are terrorized and deprives them of the opportunity to escape.

Many excellent studies have revealed how bullying thrives if teachers accept it as an inevitable part of playground life, especially where boys are concerned. Boys are more likely to bully if they have been physically beaten at home, if they are extravert in personality, and if they are failing educationally. But it turns out that there is nothing inevitable about bullying in school.

As studies such as those carried out by Dan Olweus in Norway and Peter Smith in the UK have shown, if education authorities make it clear that bullying is unacceptable, if head teachers and teachers are committed to its eradication and, above all, if children who are themselves bullied or who know of others who are bullied are empowered to act to stop it, then the problem can be markedly reduced in frequency. This occurs when there is a social disapproval of bullying among pupils and it is made easy for students to let teaching staff know anonymously when it is occurring. Of course, it is important their information is acted on effectively. Effectiveness involves good supervision by staff of all playground areas where episodes might occur and action to confront bullying children and their parents when it is detected. Some schools have found it helpful to arrange meetings with a staff member present between the parents of the bullied and the bullying students. But it is the empowerment of students themselves that is the single most important ingredient of success in reduction of bullying. No one knows better than bullied children and their classmates what is going on. No one is more motivated to do something about it than they are. The problem only persists because they do not have the power to stop it.

9.5.11 School Councils

The establishment of School Councils, again recommended in the 2001 Government Green Paper, 'Building on Success' is a further step that can be taken to provide students with a sense of responsibility. It is not known how many schools in the UK have such Councils, but surveys carried out for the

NSPCC and by Lynne Davies in the University of Birmingham suggest that most secondary schools and a small number of primary schools have one. Usually students from each year are elected to the Council by their peers. Meetings occur anything from twice a term to every week. They mostly occur in curriculum time, but are often in the lunch break or after school. A teacher usually attends, and in about three quarters of schools this is either the head teacher or deputy head teacher or both. Items discussed are many and varied. They include canteen matters, uniform, the state of the toilets, charities to be supported, the school environment, school rules, bullying policies, staff appointments, homework, timing of course work, discipline, and bullying policies.

Nearly all School Councils have ways of feeding back matters discussed and recommendations both to the student body and to the teaching staff. This is vital if the Council is to be effective. In a very small number of cases student representatives attend governors' meetings. Some teachers and some students have negative views on School Councils. Teachers may see them as taking up valuable curriculum time and are worried that damaging criticism of teachers will take place. Occasionally, students themselves feel little is accomplished by the Councils which are just talking shops, dominated by the most articulate, bossy students. The existence of some School Councils is indeed tokenistic. They provide a talking shop, but no one in authority takes the slightest notice what is said. This tends to occur when there is no support or only half-hearted support for the Council from governors, parents, and management. Without such support, suggestions made even by a well-functioning Council will only be laughed at.

But overwhelmingly the reaction of students, teachers, and head teachers is warmly enthusiastic. Ofsted inspectors are said to be 'invariably' positive about School Councils. The benefits are thought to be improvements in behaviour and discipline, ensuring students' views are accorded more respect, removing a 'them and us' ethos in the school, reducing school exclusions, sharing problems, and allowing the expression of innovative ideas. School Councils can be made to work in schools situated in deprived areas with high levels of disadvantage and disruptive pupils as well as those in more affluent localities.

9.5.12 Empowering by helping to run the school as part of work experience

I have already discussed ways in which secondary school students can be and indeed already are given work experience in the outside world through links with businesses and primary schools. Here I shall just refer to work experience within the school.

Those who visit a number of different schools often remark on the different ways they can be treated by students. In some schools, a student will volunteer to help you find your way to the person you are looking for and indeed often escort you there. In others one is completely ignored. Students in well-functioning schools see themselves as taking responsibility for creating an image for their school as a helpful, friendly place. There is every reason why such behaviour should be extended so that schools can become places where students learn work as well as study habits by taking responsibility for tasks the school needs to have carried out. Most schools run on extraordinarily small administrative and service staff. Older students could be involved, for example, in assisting in the work of the school office generally, in helping to answer some of the more routine bureaucratic enquiries local authorities make of schools, in helping to keep the school litter-free, and in assisting in the serving of school meals. Such an approach would doubtless raise the anxieties of the unions, but these could perhaps be overcome if the approach involved supplementing existing staff rather than replacing them. Further, work experience within the school would be a great deal easier to organize than in the outside world. Indeed, students themselves could help in the organization.

9.5.13 Empowering students in schools in 'challenging circumstances'

A school must surely be a place in which young people and teachers feel safe, in which, in the last resort, teachers can exercise their authority without being challenged, and in which, in short, there is an atmosphere of purpose and order. Most schools in the UK are already such places, but there is a significant number, almost entirely situated in inner city areas, in which this is clearly not the case. These are schools euphemistically termed by government departments as in 'challenging circumstances'.

In these schools, teachers cannot make themselves heard; they are at serious risk of being punched by students; most of them have indeed been attacked on at least one and often several occasions, and lessons are constantly interrupted by bickering, squabbling, and name-calling between students, or by attention-seeking behaviour. Students frequently bring weapons, especially knives, into school. Not surprisingly, teachers stay in such schools for relatively short periods, teacher recruitment is difficult or impossible, results in public examinations are abysmal, local parents do not want to send their children, and school rolls fall.

Such schools are frightening places for students, teachers, and parents. Yet their existence makes up part of the experience of a significant number of teenage young people today, an experience that is abusive to both students and teachers. Such schools are so depressing and the sense of failure within them seems so pervasive that it seems impossible they could ever change. But change they can. In the Department for Education and Employment policy document, Schools Plus, a number of examples are given of failing schools being turned around, so that they become unexpectedly successful, becoming popular with parents and prospective students, retaining staff, and obtaining distinctly better examination results.

The stories describing the turnaround of such schools share many common elements. Firm leadership from the head teacher and other senior teachers, consistency in disciplinary matters with zero tolerance of poor behaviour, and refusal to tolerate bullying are important factors. A clear focus on achievement in learning with study support programmes, consistency in homework, and marking are central features. Providing out of ordinary school hours activities such as breakfast clubs for parents and students to meet teachers informally, lunchtime clubs and homework clubs, use of increased resources to employ administrative staff to release teachers from spending their time form-filling, together with the development of links with businesses in the local community, all contribute to production of change.

The gloss or 'spin' put on these measures is that they involve the empowerment of teachers, and, of course, this is the case. But at least as importantly, and much less often mentioned, is the fact that they also empower the students, usually a majority and often a large majority, who want to learn and only need to be given the opportunity to do so. It would be futile to try to introduce many of the measures to empower students that I have mentioned earlier in this chapter. But once the school has been 'turned around', and students empowered to engage in learning the introduction of initiatives such as, school councils, is likely to prevent back-sliding into chaos.

9.5.14 Empowering the learner by meeting individual needs: the challenge

Skilled teachers rightly pride themselves on being able to meet the diverse needs of all the students in a classroom. The best do wonders in this respect, but the feedback from a large proportion of students, when asked about their school experience (some of it reported earlier in this chapter), strongly suggests that often they do not feel their individual needs are met.

The phrase 'special educational need' is usually used to describe those 10–20% of students who are suffering from some sort of disability, whether this be physical, emotional, or related to a learning problem. The fact is that *all* children and young people have special educational needs. They are all individuals with their own unique backgrounds and capacities. It is hardly surprising, given the diversity of genetic material and the great range of their experiences, this should be the case. Diversity derives from different facets of physical development, intelligence, personality, and experience.

If one looks at a photograph of a class of 13-year-olds, probably the first impression is of the enormous *variation in their physical development*. In general, the girls are taller than the boys. While some girls are, in their appearance, fully developed mature young women, looking more like average 16-year-olds, others have hardly begun to show any breast development. The same is true of boys though this is less physically obvious. A similar situation holds in intellectual development. Much is made of the fact that, in all aspects of their intelligence, girls are, on average, slightly more advanced than boys. But these sex differences are far less important than the *wide range of intellectual development* in the whole student population. While some 13-year-olds are at a stage of mature intellectual development of the average 16-year-old, others, quite apart from those with moderate or severe learning difficulties, will be more like average nine-year-olds. The ingenuity of teachers and those who devise curricula in different subjects is stretched to the limits to cater for such diverse levels of ability in age-segregated classrooms. When, for the purposes of learning in classrooms, students are strictly divided by age, teachers are faced with a virtually impossible task. Meeting such different needs within a single classroom is as difficult as it would be to fit the same pair of shoes on a group of twenty 14-year-olds.

Each year there are more successes in public examinations, normally taken by 16-year-olds, in the early teen years. It is now not at all uncommon for 13- and 14-year-olds to notch up several passes at GCSE and even 'A' levels. This has been happening in independent schools for many years. Now educationists are looking to ensure more generally that bright students are not held back by the needs of the majority and that those with special talents have them catered for. The teaching profession, while naturally concerned that the needs of less able students might be ignored, now accepts, as, for the first time, does the government, that boredom is a major problem for bright students in Years 10 and 11 of secondary schools. We should not be surprised that 13- and 14-year-olds can cope at this level. Indeed, before long, one can expect earlier achievement in public examinations to be no longer newsworthy. This will not be unexpected, for this is exactly what psychologists studying the development of intelligence would have predicted.

Diversity of *emotional maturity* is even less obvious than diversity of intellectual maturity in the school situation, yet it is becoming increasingly clear that it is relevant to success and failure in learning, especially in learning about relationships. The 14-year-old girl who can shrug off remarks made by a sarcastic teacher or rejection by a girlfriend who has started to go out with boys has less to learn about relationships than one who cannot deal with loss or disappointment without becoming deeply depressed or angrily out of control when faced with the same experiences.

Secondary students bring with them into school a set of extraordinarily *different experiences*, leading to different needs. Some will come from chaotic homes and will be crying out for firm discipline and strong external controls. Others will live in highly ordered homes and will benefit from the freedom to test boundaries and exercise their creative imaginations. Some will have supportive parents who have time to help with homework. Other supportive parents will just be too busy keeping the family afloat financially to give such help. Yet other parents will think school a waste of time and take little or no interest in whether homework is done or not. Some will live in homes where there is a quiet, private place for a student to do homework. Others will have to try to do their homework in a room in which adults are watching television and young children are trying to get to sleep.

The different backgrounds from which children come are reflected in what we know about their social circumstances. About one in five teenagers now live in families headed by a lone parent. A smaller, but not insignificant number, live with two unmarried parents. That means less than four in five have two parents 'in charge'. When discussions about the importance of marriage occur, this will mean a significant minority will feel different from the rest. About one in three 14-year-olds have experimented with cannabis: two in three have not. Information about the effects of cannabis in drug education lessons will have very different meanings for the two groups. About two in five 11–16-year-olds have part-time jobs: three in five do not. Apart from four or five DIY manuals, some children have no books at home; others will virtually have whole libraries. More and more 15-year-olds have access to the Internet, but even by the year 2002 more than half do not. Access to the Internet makes a vast difference to the knowledge store on which a student can draw. Then again, the degree of emotional turbulence in families varies widely. Some young people come to school preoccupied with the chaos and violence they have left behind at home. They may be worried their mothers will be brutally attacked while they are away or afraid an older brother will take an overdose of drugs. For others, their contented, well-ordered lives will make such events unthinkable.

9.5.15 Meeting diverse learning needs: the Internet

Many of the measures I have already outlined will go some way to meet the challenge of diversity. Interactive learning and student mentoring can both play a part, but there are many other approaches. The technology dot.com bubble may have burst, but the world of computers has already changed and will continue both to transform the process of learning and break the monopoly of information previously enjoyed by academics in universities and schools. How should teachers react to the fact that bright students in Year 9 can now obtain so much factual information from the Internet for their History and Geography essays in a single evening that will not be familiar to their teachers.

Computers have already entered the classroom. It will not be long before they have taken classrooms over. When each student has access to an individual computer with access to the Internet and an individual email address, the opportunities for active learning will have immeasurably increased. There is already a vast range of interactive software devised to enable students to learn at their own pace, receive feedback on their own performance far more rapidly than is the case when this depends on individual time being found with a teacher.

These innovatory teaching techniques have all been evaluated and found to increase motivation of students and enhance their performance. But so far they have only been employed in relatively small, often short-lived projects. The challenge is to introduce them into the mainstream where they could have a major impact in reducing the number of disaffected students as well as further improving the performance of the majority.

It should not be imagined that the introduction of IT will reduce the need for an increase in the size of the teaching force that diversity of need demands. The Internet provides information, but does not tell the user how to process the material. Using information is a much more complicated task than accessing it, and for this teachers are indispensable. The use of IT does empower students by giving them direct access to information that would not otherwise be available to them. But the presence of teachers is necessary to maximize the empowerment IT provides. Fortunately, with the employment of learning support assistants, the government has taken on the need for personal tutoring in subjects such as Mathematics and Physics in which there are major teacher shortages.

9.5.16 Empowerment requires well-maintained buildings, books, and computers

How can students feel good about themselves when society, by depriving them of decent surroundings and adequate equipment, makes it clear it does not value them? The UK school building programme has been neglected over decades. The grotty, poorly maintained buildings young people attend each day are powerful evidence of the lack of interest the state has shown in secondary age children. The amount of money schools have to spend on books and other necessary equipment is derisory. If they are to make full use of modern technology, all secondary school children over the age of 14 need a personal computer at school, with their own email address.

9.5.17 Initiation into young adulthood: the school's role

In the last chapter of this book, I suggest it would be preferable if those in their teen years were regarded as in the earliest part of young adulthood, rather than that they were still either children or in some adolescent no man's land between childhood and adulthood. This would mean that the learning experience of the 14–18-year-old would be seen less as a continuation of childhood schooling (though, of course, it would still partly be that) and more as the start of self-motivated, lifelong learning throughout the whole of adulthood. Preparation for public examinations beginning at 14 years for those taken at 16 years and then at 18 years would be seen, not as marking the end of childhood, but as the first of a series of nationally accredited courses for qualifications that individuals would have to take to demonstrate their competence in their area of work or in new fields throughout their working lives.

If it were generally accepted that 14 years or the beginning of Key Stage 4, marked the beginning of adult life, some schools might regard it as appropriate for there to be some public acknowledgement of the fact. A ceremony, to which parents would be invited, initiating 14-year-olds at the beginning of the relevant school year into new rights and new responsibilities. Rights might relate to some aspects of dress and school uniform (either the right not to wear uniform or to wear some differentiating mark), the right to wear personal jewellery, access to particular study rooms, and eligibility to serve on the School Council. Responsibilities might include mentoring of younger children, more autonomy in studying at school, and an expectation of help in keeping the school premises free of litter. The linking of rights with responsibilities could do much to bring those in their teens into better contact with the wider world.

Chapter 10

Leisure and work

During the last hundred years, leisure and, to a lesser extent school, have replaced work in the way young people in their teens spend their time. But, having given them so much leisure time, the adult world has failed to provide for it, complaining about the way the young spend it, but largely leaving them powerless to do anything about it themselves. Of course, the young do fill their time especially if, in their mid and late teens, they are completely dedicated to working for public examinations. But this leaves most of those in their early teens and many of those in their late teens with a time vacuum, often filled, as we shall see, only with empty boredom.

10.1 How satisfied are the teens with their leisure activities?

The large sample of Glasgow 13- and 14-year-olds described in the last chapter and studied by Jackie Gordon and Gillian Grant were asked what they felt about their time outside school. These were some of the replies:

I feel very tired today. But I feel tired every day, very depressed and bored. All me and my friends do is walk about the streets. There is nothing in X … for us to do. Sometimes I get very angry about having my own kids and bringing them up in X … When I get angry I get awful crabby and take everything out on my friends. Everyone thinks I am going daft because of the way I am going, but it's not me, it's the place I am living. Today I feel down, I feel as if the world is going round and round and I am going to fall off.

There is nothing to do around my bit. You can either stay in or walk around the streets doing nothing. If you even play football somewhere you get told to go away.

I feel as though there is nothing to look forward to as it is so boring at night. I live in … so it is not as though they are going to build a youth club or something because they think it is all drugs there or bad people. If there were more things to do more youngsters would stay out of crime.

I love to go out and have a laugh, but me and my pals can't even walk along the road without the police booking us—and it is for nothing—I think they are just bored too!

This is not just a Scottish view. A similar picture emerged from interviews carried out by Anita Franklin and Nicola Madge with 11–16-year-olds in

Lewisham, London. When asked what they would do to make things better for young people if they were Mayor of Lewisham, the responses frequently revolved round better leisure facilities:

> Please do something about our area because we are all classed as delinquents but we are not. We want somewhere to go. Thank you (female aged 14).
>
> No things for teenagers to do after school—there is nowhere to go you just hang around the streets (female aged 14).
>
> Young people are getting bored, that's why we do graffiti, we are bored, we need something to do (aged 10).
>
> There's loads of violence in D ... — they ain't got nothing to do.

The lack of things to do outside school or College is now widely experienced as a source of serious dissatisfaction among young people in their teens. Unfortunately there are no very satisfactory surveys documenting the extent of the dissatisfaction, and we have to rely on the local studies such as those I have just quoted. All the same, Tim Gill of the Children's Play Council, a national organization concerned with leisure activities of those in their teens as well as play for younger children, confirms there is a strong and widespread consensus among youth workers, teachers, and parents that the level of dissatisfaction among young people in their teens with their out of school experience is considerable.

10.2 Why are those in their teens so dissatisfied with what happens out of school?

10.2.1 Changes in the balance of work and leisure

A hundred years ago, as we saw in the last chapter, in the early years of the twentieth century, nearly all young people between 13 and 18 years old were in full-time work. Even most young people in the middle classes finished their education round about the age of 14 years old. Only a few went on to further education in school and fewer still to universities. The boys went to work in offices, in the family business or shop, or on the family farm. Boys of the labouring classes were all at work by this age in manual jobs in factories or in the fields. Whatever their social class, most girls were at home helping with domestic tasks, though many were now entering offices or shops or, in the labouring classes, especially in the north of England were factory workers. Gradually compulsory education took over the teens. As we shall see in the last chapter, compulsory education to 14 years was introduced in 1919, to 15 years with the 1944 Education Act, and to 16 years in 1972. Since the 1970s the proportion of young people aged 16–18 years in full-time education has increased steadily, so that only about one in ten 16–17-year-olds were in full-time work at the beginning of the twenty-first century. Over 40% now go on to the University and the government aims for a target of 50% by 2006. The result of this dramatic change is that, over a hundred years, in the life of the teens, exhausting but productive and paid work has almost entirely been taken over by school, college, and free time. For some young people, especially those with less academic ability or interest, this has not been a happy transformation.

10.2.2 Changes making home a less hospitable place after school

Up to the 1970s, when those in their teens came home from school, there was often one parent in the home after school or in the holidays. This meant that home was not experienced as an empty place, but somewhere one could touch base, have a chat, or drink a cup of tea together. Now it is much more common for both parents to be working and out of the house. Of course, young people, especially as they move into mid and late adolescence will see their friends as better company than their parents, but parents have always previously been a fall back when other company is not available. Now that is usually not an option.

10.2.3 Consumerism

The free market economy has improved the lives of many of those in their teens. It has been at least partly responsible for the greater prosperity of families with children of this age. Without market competition it is at least uncertain whether the various technical advances of the twentieth century, at first radio and television, and then videos, computers, video games, and mobile phones, would have been made to make so widely available. All of these have enriched the lives of the young as well as those of adults. The young are now generally much better clothed than they were. Of course, not all young people have benefited to the same degree, but even those in low income families virtually always have access to radio, television and video recorders, and many have mobile phones.

The young are now big business. Louis Barfe calculated that in 1997 in the UK, the under-16s market alone was worth £16.18 billion. A more recent survey by ChildWise, probably the main agency providing information to those wishing to market to the teens, reports that almost all children over nine years of age have money of their own to spend. ChildWise states that the combined direct spending power of the 5–16-year age group amounts to around £2.3 billion per year in the UK, mostly by those at the upper end of the age group. However, much more is spent by parents on their children, especially on clothes, including footwear. It is estimated that the average amount spent on clothes per month in 2002 for the 11–16-year age group was £31.70 on clothes and £29.40 on footwear. For this age group the largest item of direct expenditure was on music/CDs, with lesser amounts on magazines/comics, crisps/snacks, and sweets/chocolates.

In addition, and, for those in the market probably more importantly, teenage children have some influence on a whole range of purchases made by adults, including their home computers, televisions, DVDs, cars, cameras, in some cases doubtless the houses they buy. The total figure for expenditure in the United States for which those in their teens have some influence has been put at $520 billion.

The main market sectors for those in their early and mid-teens are food and drink; clothing and footwear; books and magazines; toys, games, and sports goods. From the early teens, suppliers target the young themselves rather than their parents, as it is the young who make the purchasing decisions. The youth sector of the market is growing faster than that for younger children. In the mid-nineties it grew by 26% over a four-year period and, although the figures are not available, it is highly likely there has been a very considerable increase since that time. Much of the increase has come about through character licensing, the linking of goods to television, sporting, or other stars with considerable hikes on the price of branded items recommended by favourite personalities.

There is no doubt that this sector of the market is thriving. We saw in Chapter 1, how the adult world discriminates against the young, but it is more than prepared to take their money! A number of questions arise from these figures. Whatever the contribution of the market in the past, to what degree does this vast level of expenditure enhance the quality of life of young people? As Alissa Quart describes in her book 'Branded: The Buying and Selling of Teenagers', the teenage market, like that of markets directed towards other age groups, operates by creating needs and desires and therefore dissatisfaction. As far as the young are concerned, this mainly revolves around the marketing of clothing and footwear. No sooner have they bought an item linked to the currently favourite personality, than the market is manipulated to create further demand by hyping up some other star. Nowhere is the creation of dissatisfaction so blatantly pursued. The magazines that are sold are largely vehicles for the marketing of fashion items. The pleasure they give is fleeting and, although there is a great deal to be said for fleeting pleasures, they do seem to come extremely expensive for the young and their parents.

The market may well have been responsible for many of the improvements in teenage life, but it has also become a powerful engine for the creation of dissatisfaction. In groups of young people in which the status of individuals is strongly assessed by their peers on the basis of the value of the trainers they wear and the mobile phones they own, those in disadvantaged circumstances, especially if they are living among a generally wealthier group, are likely to feel deprived and frustrated.

10.2.4 Government and local authority inaction

As education has gradually taken over the life of the teens, central government and local authorities have largely ignored the large tracts of time that have, as a result, become available to the young. Until recently the free time or leisure needs of this age group have not been adequately investigated and conse-quently there has been no possibility of meeting them. While there has been a significant increase in after school activities on school premises in infant and primary schools, this has occurred to a much smaller extent in relation to sec-ondary schools and colleges of further education.

10.3 Effects of ignoring the free time or leisure needs of the young

The quotations with which this chapter began, provide eloquently expressed evidence of the problems that have arisen. It is sometimes suggested, even by mental health professionals, that boredom and depression are just a natural part of adolescence or growing up. But, as we saw in Chapter 1, this is a myth, like so many other beliefs about the age group. Many young people of this age are capable of making their own entertainment or their desire to study and ambition to obtain good grades is so great that how to spend leisure time is not a problem for them. But many are poorly equipped to find things to do when they are bored. If their friends are not available to 'hang out' with, they may put on a video, watch TV, or play a computer game, but if they find this unsatisfy-ing, they are lost to know what to do. Depression is not the same as boredom, as we saw in Chapter 4, but if there are other reasons for a teenager to become depressed, boredom can act as an extra trigger, with distressing consequences.

The other main consequence of a lack of leisure facilities is very much in the public eye. It is one important cause of 'temporary' delinquency, the type of antisocial behaviour, I describe in Chapter 5, that is shown by young people in their teens who are not particularly disobedient in childhood and do not offend later in adult life. It has been shown that if 14- or 15-year-old are under stress, the existence of places for them to go to play sport or pursue some other interest, will play some part in protecting them from getting into trouble with the police.

10.4 **Changing patterns of leisure during the teens**

The publication Social Focus on Young People provides much interesting information on the way the young spend their time. The average 13–14-year-old now spends about 40 h (30%) of his or her waking time at school or doing homework. About 10% or two hours a day is spent on what might be called survival tasks, like eating, washing etc. So 60% of an average teenager's day is 'free time'. This percentage varies from country to country. In some South-East Asian countries, such as Hong Kong and Singapore, many teenagers have only 10% of free time, because there is so much emphasis on education, school hours are longer, and more time is spent on homework or private tuition. Free time also varies from teenager to teenager in the UK and the USA. Some will spend much more time on study, much more like the south east Asia situation. Others spend less time studying, though few will spend much less than half their time in this way, as compulsory school and homework take up so much of it.

From newspaper headlines one might think that teenagers spend all their free time hanging around on street corners waiting to rob old ladies, breaking into cars, or dealing in drugs. The reality is very different. How do British adolescents spend the leisure time these days? Surveys suggest that there is a progression of leisure pursuits during adolescence. The 12–13-year-olds engage more in 'organized' leisure such as club sports (when they are available) and after-school activities; the 14–15-year-olds move to 'casual' leisure activities such as hanging around with friends.

John Balding of the Exeter Schools Health Education Unit regularly reports the results of an annual survey in which information is obtained about the daily lives of 14–15-year-olds throughout England. Over a half, spend more than one hour watching television each day and about one in six spend more than three hours a day this way. About one in three boys and one in twenty girls spend more than an hour playing computer games. So far no survey information is available on the amount of time spent by adolescents on the Internet, but this must be rapidly increasing.

When asked what they have done on the previous day, about one in ten 14–15-year-olds had watched a video. Two in three boys and four in five girls had listened to recorded music, though probably much time spent listening to music was taken up with other activities undertaken at the same time. One in eight had played a musical instrument. About a half of the adolescents surveyed had met with friends. Two in five had read a magazine, but only one in eight had read a book for enjoyment. About half had spent time caring for pets. Half the boys and a quarter of the girls had played some sort of sport.

About a third of both boys and girls had had an alcoholic drink at home, and about one in five at a friend's home. One in eight had consumed alcohol at a disco, club or party and one in ten in a pub or bar. One in five had drunk alcohol in a public place, but about half had not consumed alcohol at all in the previous week. In general, a national picture emerges then of adolescents in their early and mid-teen years spending a lot of their time outside school at home, doing homework, watching television, listening to recorded music, reading magazines, and playing computer games. Less time, but all the same a substantial amount, is spent watching videos, reading, and caring for pets. Out of the home, meeting with friends is easily the most common activity, and this usually happens in homes or on the street. But the pattern can vary greatly.

Sam is 13 years old and lives in a deprived area of east London. Her parents are both working, but in low income jobs, her father as a security guard and her mother as a cleaner. She has a 16-year-old sister. The family live in a two bedroom flat and Sam shares a room with her sister. When she comes home from school, she tries to do her homework, but her sister who has dropped out of education but has not found a job, is likely to be playing music at high volume and not much homework gets done. Sam does have a mobile and rings round her friends. Few of them live in places where they can hang out together in peace and safety. The local park, where they do tend to go, is unsafe because of muggings linked to drug dealing. There is another park nearby, but it is an unpleasant place to be because of the dog mess everywhere. The situation is the same at weekends. Sam does not think much of the leisure facilities provided by her local authority.

Nicky is a 13-year-old girl living about 5 miles away from Sam, in the north of London. Her parents are comfortably off as both of them work full-time, her father as a solicitor and her mother as a doctor. She also has a 16-year-old sister. The four of them live in a large four bedroom house with a garden. When she comes home from school, Nicky chills out in the kitchen with a cold drink and then goes up to her room where she puts on her CD player and completes her homework. This takes about an hour and then she begins to ring her friends to find out who is available to chat or listen to music that afternoon. All her friends live within easy and safe walking distance in the middle class district in which she lives. They all also have rooms of their own. At the weekend she, her sister, and her parents go to a health and fitness club where they have a family membership and play tennis together with friends. On Saturday mornings, she goes to her violin teacher and sometimes plays in a small youth group on Sunday mornings. Nicky has never given a thought to what her local authority provides in the way of leisure facilities.

As young people move into later adolescence, if they can afford it and have the time, they are likely to be more involved in commercialized leisure activities. The proportions spending at least part of their leisure time drinking alcohol or using drugs rapidly rises. There is also a change in where young people drink, so that by the age of 18 years, pubs or clubs are as frequently cited as places to drink as is home, which is where younger teenagers mostly drink. Young people are more likely to be regular drinkers once they are physically mature, so between 12 and 15 years sexually mature young people, probably because they are mixing more with older teenagers, drink more alcohol than those who have still not reached puberty. However, once teenagers have formed reasonably stable romantic relationships, they drink less. A Dutch study showed that even 14–18-year-olds, both boys and girls, but especially boys, drank much more alcohol if they did not have a regular friend of the opposite sex. Again though, there is great variation in how older teenagers spend their out of school time, even if they are still studying.

Jake is a 17-year-old, attending a College of Further Education in south London. His parents both work full-time from 9 am to 6 pm in different estate agencies. Jake spends from 9 am to 1 pm most days taking courses for his three 'A' levels, and on three afternoons a week he has further courses from 1.30 to 3.30 pm. He spends about two hours a day during the week and another four hours over the weekend on homework. This leaves him large slabs of time free to do what he wants and, as Jake is not particularly ambitious to do well in his exams (he has no wish to go to the University), he is not keen to do any more studying. A couple of afternoons a week after College he kicks a football around in a park with friends. He takes no other exercise. The rest of the time he spends with a mixed group about his own age, listening to music, in coffee bars or, in the evenings, in pubs. (Jake looks older than his age.) On Fridays and Saturdays he goes clubbing with his friends. He usually gets home around 2 am, and this means that most of the Saturday and Sunday mornings he spends in bed. He doesn't smoke, but binge drinks at the weekend. He is able to finance his leisure activities (including a couple of ecstasy tablets at the clubs he goes to) as well as some of his clothes purchases (his parents give the rest) from the £10 a week he gets from his father and £5 from his mother, together with another £20 a week (£4 an hour) working as a checkout clerk or stacking shelves on Saturday afternoons from noon to 5 pm.

Tom is 17 years old and is following a similar course at a College of Further Education in a deprived area in the north-east of England. His mother has a part-time job as a secretary, but his father, a steel worker who was made redundant 10 years ago, is unemployed. Tom has a younger sister at school and the family income is low. Tom's course takes up about the same amount of time as Jake's, but he spends the rest of his time very differently. He has a care assistant job in a residential home for the elderly for 30 hours a week, working from 5 pm in the late afternoon to 11 pm in the evenings for five days a week on weekdays and for five hours a week on Saturdays during the day, so he earns around £120 a week. He goes to a pub with friends on Saturday evenings. However, he spends little on clothes or on any other form of entertainment. He has a lie in on Sunday mornings and does homework on Sunday afternoon. He is able to give his mother around £80 a week from his earnings and this is an essential contribution to the family income, as without it there would not be sufficient to pay the gas, electricity, and food bills.

The difference in the lives of these two young men is substantial. Jake's way of life, with its emphasis on relatively expensive leisure pursuits, is far more common in the UK at the present time. Most of his entertainment is centred round activities specifically designed for people very close to his age, so there is no way he can mix with people older than himself. He is too young to be a member of the local health club, so he has very little opportunity to keep fit. There are no opportunities for him to spend his time in any creative activities even if he wanted to. Tom does not have the time or money to engage in any leisure activities of this sort anyway, but if he did they would not be available in his area.

10.5 The leisure needs of the young in their teen years

What young people, especially girls in their early and mid-teens say they want more than anything else out of school or college hours is a place to go that is safe and clean where they can hang out with friends. Obviously girls like Nicky are not likely to express this need because they already have such a place, but most young people of their age are not as lucky as she is. Boys of this age will want the same but also somewhere they can kick a ball around or play a proper team game. Ideally they would prefer their place to hang out to be out of doors because of the greater sense of freedom this provides, but British weather being as it is, it is probably more realistic to think in terms of under cover or inside accommodation for at least six months of the year.

At the present time, especially in big cities, the shopping mall is increasingly becoming the place where the young 'hang out'. The fact that the main purpose of the mall is to encourage expenditure makes it an unsatisfactory place for this to occur. Addictive slot machines and the display of usually unattainable branded goods in close proximity creates social and personal problems for young people rather than sorting them out.

Safe 'hanging out' is not the only activity the young of this age wish for. Many would also like to be able to pursue an interest in art, drama, music, or some other creative activity. Quite a number would be glad of the opportunity to spend time practicing and learning more computer skills. Some, especially but not only boys, would like much more rigorous training or coaching in a sport, not necessarily football. Schools, with their emphasis on academic subjects, are often not able to provide such experience. In any case, many young people would like to engage in creative activity in a more relaxed atmosphere than is possible at school.

10.6 **What needs to happen**

Although it would be preferable if there had been more and better quality consultations carried out with young people, the results of surveys carried out by the government and by a number of local authorities are reasonably clear-cut. They make it clear what young people would like to be made available out of school hours. Their wishes seem entirely reasonable. What needs to happen now is for the money and the people to make it all happen. Because successive governments have largely removed the right of young people to work (though I shall have more to say about this later in this chapter), it is not reasonable to expect the young to pay for the changes that are needed. On the other hand, it would be highly desirable if, as far as possible, extra staff needed were drawn from the ranks of the young themselves. Certainly young people should be prominent in any group, planning improved youth facilities in a local area.

The first requirement is for existing space to be made safe and clean. Young people in their teens who are, as I suggest in other chapters, to all intents and purposes young though inexperienced adults, do not want to be supervised, but they do rely on the older adult population to make both public parks and the streets leading to youth clubs safe places to be. This means that they have to be clear of drug dealing and drug addicts, the main causes of seriously violent crime in our cities today. I discussed different ways this might be achieved in Chapter 7. The young could certainly be involved in keeping public areas safe and clean.

Linked to this need for space outside the home is the need for those in their teens to have control over some personal private space in their own home, basically a room to themselves. It is already accepted that housing standards are not met unless young people of this age are either in rooms of their own or sharing with others of the same sex, but this is not really sufficient. The sex of a sibling does not affect the need of a young person to have some personal space. Just because a young person has a same sex sibling should not deprive them of a room to themselves.

Although, as a group, young people of this age give priority to the need for space to hang out with their friends, a large number of them wish to spend at least some of their time out of school hours engaged in one or more focused activities. For this activity, whether it be music, art, creative writing, a sport or keep fit exercising, they need good equipment and people with some expertise to guide them. At the present time, apart from the very privileged such as Nicky, most young people are excluded from such activity either because the cost is beyond them or because there is no place they can go that is near enough. For the very talented young musician, artist, footballer, gymnast, or swimmer, there will be opportunities laid on for the gifted, but many who do not have such outstanding talent would enjoy the opportunity to participate in such activity outside the school setting. Some would be discovered to have remarkable, untapped potential if only they had the chance to show it. Indeed very talented young people could be part of those providing the expertise.

Young people in general like to be in groups of their own age. So do we all, though perhaps not to the same degree. Is it possible that this need, young people to huddle together, arises partly because of the fact that they feel 'got at' and stigmatized by older people who expect nothing but trouble from them? In any case, it seems undesirable that young people should be so separate from the rest of the population. Leisure activities and lifelong learning provide opportunities for some degree of mixing of the ages. In some cities, for example, older people are brought together with the young so that they can learn computer skills from 13- and 14-year-olds. Music groups, chess clubs, and some sporting activities are other opportunities for older adults and the young to learn from each other.

10.7 **Work in the teens**

For many young people in their early and mid-teens, school, as we shall see in the last chapter, though changes are taking place to alter this situation, remains a pretty disempowering experience. The opportunity to work part-time and earn some money of their own could give them a degree of independence they otherwise lack. For most young people in their teens, paid employment takes up a relatively small part of their free time. This has, of course, not always been the case. Until 150 years ago, it was assumed that it was acceptable for children to work well before they reached their teens. Then, in the first half of the nineteenth century, descriptions of the appalling conditions in which young children worked, especially in the factories of the north of England, stimulated the passage of protective legislation. Such legislation was mainly aimed at children under the age of 13 years, and there was no attempt to limit the work of young people over this age.

All the same, public disapproval of young people in their mid-teens working gradually increased throughout the nineteenth century. The need for unskilled labour in the First World War predictably resulted in a change of attitude. There was much less disapproval of teen employment. Indeed, as indicated in Chapter 2, even the professional view changed. Work was seen by psychologists as character building and necessary for satisfactory adolescent development. After the Second World War, full employment continued until the late 1970s, but the rate of unemployment in the general population first gradually and then sharply rose to a peak in the mid-eighties.

At this point, it became widely accepted that it was desirable for the young to continue in education beyond the compulsory school leaving age. This occurred for a variety of reasons. The need for a work force that was better educated became apparent. It also became clear that the working class young were becoming seriously disadvantaged because they did not stay on in education. This was increasing social and economic inequalities. A more cynical view is that the young were contributing to high unemployment figures. This was politically embarrassing, so successive governments produced policies giving strong encouragement to those in their mid and late teens to remain in full-time education or join training schemes, some of which were quite unsatisfactory.

10.8 Attitudes to teen employment

With employment opportunities now extremely variable throughout the UK, the attitude of the adult population to young people working is divided. On the one hand, even part-time work is seen as exposing the young to exploitation and as harmful to educational achievement. Alternatively, it is seen as desirable for young people to earn at least some of their own money and not be dependent on the provision of pocket money from parents or, later, from state benefits.

In general, parents and the public at large seem to approve of young people in their early and mid-teens working, while the teaching profession is negative in its attitude, seeing time spent in employment as a distraction from homework and study. Parents who have used an authoritative approach to bringing up their children (see Chapter 3) often try to enhance their independence by ensuring that the pocket money they provide does not cover what might be regarded as luxuries. If their children want more than the basic extras, they have to earn the money for them themselves. Such an approach is made more difficult when other parents are lashing out large sums every week or on demand, but many young people appreciate the fact that luxuries have to be earned and that they can gain this from their work experience.

The young themselves, as Virginia Morrow suggests, mainly work to earn money so that they can participate in society as consumers. They look for paid employment if they feel their parents cannot afford to give them the money they need to make purchases that will help to establish their identities as members of their age group. Thus they work to obtain what might seem to the adult world to be the latest consumer luxuries, but seem to them totally necessary so that they can fully belong to the group of young people with whom they identify. A relatively small number of young people of this age, like 17-year-old Tom, described earlier in this chapter, living in low-income families, need to work to bring family income above survival level. In fact, although young people living in poverty often want to help to contribute to the family income, they are actually less likely to be in work than those in more affluent families because they are usually living in areas of high unemployment where they cannot find work.

10.9 **A moderate amount of work benefits the young**

The evidence that young people are harmed by the experience of taking on paid employment is very limited or non-existent. To some extent, the reverse is the case. Unfortunately, most of the studies come from the United States where the situation is different because a much higher proportion of young people of this age are in part-time employment. All the same, it is interesting that American findings, as summarized by psychologists Jeylan Mortimer and Monica Johnson, suggest that young people who work less than 20 hours a week or at 'low intensity' do better in all sorts of ways than those who work longer hours and those who do not work at all. Young people who work at 'low intensity' are more motivated in their schoolwork, have higher academic self-esteem, and get better grades. There is some concern that those young people who work might establish an adult lifestyle too early, for example, by settling into cohabiting relationships prematurely, but this is not the case. Following up these young people into adulthood, it turns out that 'low intensity' young workers have a better educational outcome and find it easier to settle into occupations than the other two groups. So rather than harming young people, low intensity work seems to confer benefit. In contrast, though the findings are complex and differ depending on which measures are examined, not working or working at high intensity is followed by less satisfactory outcomes. So part-time work provides the young with a supplement to their pocket money, and conveys other benefits. It is also, of course, one way of introducing the young to the world of work.

10.10 **How much do those in their teens work and what do they do?**

The fact that young people in their early and mid-teens have had to attend school has not deterred many from finding paid part-time employment well before they leave school. The government publication mentioned earlier in this chapter, Social Focus on Young People, reports that in 1997, one in four 11–16-year-olds had a current term-time job and one in five had had a job during the last summer holiday. Most of these were aged 14–16 years old, though quite a few 11–13-year-olds also have jobs. Overall, 38% of the 11–16-year-olds had had a job some time in the last year. Once they reach the age of 16 years, 70% are in full-time and a further 15% are in part-time education and training. However, a high proportion of those in full-time education are also in some form of employment, usually part-time, and an even higher proportion of those in part-time education are also working.

This trend to continue working despite being in full-time education continues for those who go to university. Usually it is earning money to supplement grants and paying off debts that motivates nearly half those in full-time education to find employment. Most of the jobs are in the distribution trade or in hotels or restaurants.

Many young people work for little or no money. They may be helping, for example, in family businesses, such as sandwich bars or small restaurants. As we saw in Chapter 3, a smaller number, but still as many as 70 000 in the UK, work unpaid as 'young carers', looking after dependent relatives, especially parents, grandparents, and disabled brothers and sisters

The paid jobs young people of this age obtain vary very considerably. They are most likely to be repetitive and boring, for example, stacking shelves in supermarkets. Baby-sitting, gardening, delivering newspapers, waiting at tables, or doing kitchen work in restaurants can be more interesting, but there are negative aspects to this type of work. They provide little opportunity for learning new skills. Often they involve working only with other young people in almost entirely age-segregated work settings, so they do not bring the young into contact with older people. It could be said that they provide experience that enables young people to cope with boredom, monotony, and their own anger and frustration at having to cope with unreasonable pressures. Doubtless many young people would say they get quite enough of this sort of experience at school.

Clearly the jobs young people obtain do not in any way allow them to fulfil their employment potential. In the last section of this chapter, I give some examples of the way young people in their mid-teens can achieve surprisingly well if, as has recently happened as a result of advances in communication technology, the constraints on them are lifted.

10.11 **Empowering the young to work**

The present situation regarding the employment of young people in their teens is unsatisfactory. The adult world has created a situation in which many young people of this age are exploited in very low paid jobs. Most of these are working at well below their potential. Some are working long hours at this young age in order to ensure their families rise above subsistence level. That cannot be right. Other young people of this age do not gain the valuable experience that work can provide because their parents can afford to give them large amounts of pocket money. These are denied the satisfaction of spending money they have earned themselves. Thus the area of youth employment shows all the features that characterize the way the adult world treats young people in their teens. They are exploited, infantilized, and disempowered, and often inadequately protected. What can be done?

10.12 **The law on the employment of the young**

At the present time, this is both too restrictive and not restrictive enough. It is also often completely ignored. For example, 13–15-year-olds are supposed to have a license to work, but they often don't. They are not allowed to work before 7 am or after 7 pm. This seems reasonable. Thirteen- and 14-year-olds are not supposed to work more than five hours a day and 15-year-olds no more than eight hours. That 13-year-olds should be allowed to work at all seems questionable, but eight hours a day seems a great deal for a 15-year-old, except in unusual circumstances. There is a two hours restriction on work on Sundays that most young people think is unreasonable, and they are surely right.

At the present time these laws are, as a paper prepared in 1998 by a number of UK children's organizations states 'confused, very complicated and currently fail children who work … They make little sense to working children themselves and do not reflect the reality of children's lives'. It would be helpful to have a set of agreed principles around the area of the employment of the young to which parents and teachers could subscribe.

These might include:

- Education is the paramount requirement of young people throughout their teens.

- Young people over the age of 14 years, who wish to work a reasonable number of hours a week should be empowered to do so. For young people aged over 14 years a moderate level of employment, say around 10–15 hours a week, does not interfere with educational progress. On the contrary, it enhances it and provides valuable experience.

- With this in mind, parents who give their children very generous amounts of pocket money, making it pointless for them to work, should consider whether they are denying them the opportunity to gain experience in the world of work.

♦ Children aged 13 years or under should not be allowed to work. Protective legislation should be in place to ensure they do not do paid work.

♦ As far as possible, young people should be given the opportunity in their employment to do work that has some learning or useful experience component.

♦ The young, like people of all ages, should be adequately protected against physical hazards and accidents. Their employers should be insured in case they are injured at work.

♦ Employers should require a licence to employ young people of this age.

♦ The benefit system needs to be set at a level to ensure that it is not necessary for 14–18-year-olds to work in order for their families to be able to enjoy a reasonable standard of living.

♦ If it is not practicable for a minimum wage to be set for young people of this age, at least the employer's licence should state what wages are being offered, so that the young know what they are entitled to.

♦ Through Youth Councils (see Chapter 11), young people should be consulted about their conditions of employment.

♦ These laws should also apply to the school-based work experience initiatives that I have described in the previous chapter. However, such work experience is not likely to replace paid employment among young people in their teens.

10.13 **Freeing the entrepreneurial spirit**

Finally in this discussion of teenage work, let me give some examples of what can happen when young people in their mid-teens are allowed to use their initiative in the commercial world. As the nature of work has changed, with increased opportunities for Internet trade, so there has been a growing number of teenage Internet entrepreneurs. They work, sometimes with great success, in the investment trade, developing software, and generally exploring innovative uses of the Internet.

There are a number of striking examples of young people in their teens who have made fortunes in this way. Dominic McVey discovered Viza scooters on the net and bought the European distribution rights at the age of 14. He set up his own company, Scooters UK and in 2001 was, at the age of 16 years, personally valued at £1.5 million. At the age of 15, Ben Cohen set up his own website, jewishnet.co.uk that included innovations such as the world's first cyber rabbi and a service matching Jewish customers with Jewish tradespeople. He sold this website for £300,000 in the year 2000. But these are not isolated examples of entrepreneurship in young people in their mid-teens. It is estimated that around 12% of US and UK teenagers own stocks, and a stock market advice centre, Teenanalyst, set up by a couple of adolescents, gives investment tips to around 10 000 users a month. This tendency has not passed unnoticed by Gordon Brown, the UK Chancellor of the Exchequer. In the year 2000, he made it possible for the first time, for 16- and 17-year-olds to open ISAs, or Investment Savings Accounts.

Michael Lewis, in his book 'The Future Just Happened', reports how young people of this age, by their ingenuity and entrepreneurial skill, can also provide uncomfortable insights into the way the adult business world works. In his book, Lewis describes his interviews with Jonathan Lebed, the 14-year-old who manipulated the American stock market and enraged the US Securities and Exchange Commission (SEC) by his success. Every morning, Jonathan would buy stock and post messages talking up the stock he had purchased as a best buy for small investors. During the day, he would help some of his schoolmates and indeed some of his teachers to make significant profits themselves. In the evening he would come home, note how his stocks had risen and sell them. In this way he rapidly made around $800,000 before he was hauled before the SEC and fined for blatant market manipulation. But, as Jonathan pointed out to Lewis and to his lawyers, his behaviour merely mimicked what those involved in the stock market were doing all the time.

Lewis describes the major advances that have taken place in modern technology through observing children and those in their teens and exploiting their capacity for innovative thinking. Untrammelled by preconceived ideas, they can freely associate in a manner that adults have lost to achieve creative solutions to problems that have baffled older people. He cites Nokia, the Finnish mobile phone company, as having developed text message technology by observing how young people in their teens communicated.

In fact there is no reason to idealize teenage thought processes in this way. There are plenty of examples of older people who have retained the capacity to innovate well into their sixties. But the capacities of young people in their early and mid-teens have been consistently underestimated and have only recently been liberated by the development of the Internet. Society and teens themselves would benefit if there was a more positive attitude to the idea of empowering the teens to work again.

Chapter 11

Joining up the teens again

11.1 Confusion about the teen years

In previous chapters we have seen how young people of teen age, quite contrary to the popular view, are mostly reasonably well-behaved, cheerful, equable, and studious. They find much to enjoy in their lives, especially their friendships, their leisure activities, and their family life. In support of this conclusion, a report from the Future Foundation, based on a survey of 500 representative 13–18-year-olds in the spring of 2002, concludes 'Most teenagers express broad satisfaction with their lives. The majority choose to describe their lives as happy, fun, and carefree. Much of this satisfaction stems from their lives outside of school, where they are enjoying growing freedoms .... The majority express satisfaction with their family life and enjoy a supportive relationship with their parents .... Astonishingly, a third of teenagers claim they have not argued at all with their parents in the past year'. So this is not a time of life that parents should anticipate with the fear and trembling that some of the media and indeed some professionals seem to encourage. Those in their teens who, as children, got by reasonably well can be expected to continue to do so. Some will have difficulties, but many of those who do will have been troubled since their earlier years. The teen years are not a cure for troubled behaviour; nor do they, as a general rule, cause trouble. Most parents and young people themselves can look forward to the teens as an enjoyable and rewarding time of life.

In the chapter on teenage moods and moodiness, it transpired that most young people of this age are reasonably happy most of the time. Among a minority similar in size to that in the adult population, there are significant rates of depression. Those young people with disturbed emotions are not showing trivial upset. They sometimes suffer so deeply they attempt or even very, very occasionally commit suicide. Stresses, pressures, and disappointments producing depression are, of course, different for each age group. In the teens, family arguments, loss of relationships, being bullied, and examination stresses are commonly in the background, with not being listened to, and lack of power to escape from intolerable situations or painful predicaments as common themes.

In the next chapter on conflict and antisocial behaviour, we found that most young people were well-behaved and conforming, and that the small minority who are seriously problematic have usually been showing similar serious problems since their early childhood. The disruptive behaviour they show not only affects their own lives but the lives of others, for example, making school classrooms places where useful learning just cannot occur no matter how good the teaching, or is completely ruining the lives of elderly people whom they terrorize. The much more common rebellious, but sometimes more serious antisocial behaviour of those in their teens who have been well-behaved beforehand and will be law-abiding citizens by their mid to late twenties is commonly linked to feelings of alienation in school, lack of anything much to do outside school and, more generally, to the lack of control young people of this age have over their own lives.

In the chapter discussing the sexual behaviour of young people, it became clear that, though most of those in their teens try to behave responsibly in this area of their lives, the adult world disempowers them, making it difficult for those physically mature young people who choose to have sexual relationships to do so safely, preparing them poorly for sexual experience and making it more difficult than it need be for them to use contraception. The unplanned pregnancies, sexually transmitted infections, and abusive relationships that are experienced by a minority arise at least partly because of the difficulties young people have in obtaining reliable information and in gaining access to sexual health services.

We saw in the chapter on drugs and alcohol how most young people do not abuse drugs or alcohol, but use them in an experimental fashion to achieve the results they want without significant danger. But the ready availability of illegal drugs and the laws governing possession and use mean that the young are often exposed to more danger from the criminal activities of the drug trade than from use of the drugs themselves. Despite their widespread use of both drugs and alcohol, the young are neither adequately protected nor prepared for harmful effects. A small, vulnerable minority, especially those living in deprived, crime-ridden areas, are in grave danger of developing addiction.

Because of inadequate exercise and overeating a sizeable number of young people arrive in their teens seriously overweight, having been inadequately protected against obesity in childhood. When looking at dieting behaviour, we saw how many young people eat sensibly, but that commercial pressure from the fashion trade through magazines and other media to achieve a particular body shape means that a high proportion are dissatisfied and unhappy about their appearance, and a significant minority develop anorexia. These may starve themselves to a worrying degree, very, very occasionally to the point of death.

Looking at secondary schools in Chapter 9, we found that, though many of those in their teens enjoy school and are successful there, at any rate up to the age of 16, and in practice up to the age of 18 or 19 years, a significant minority are forced to spend a large part of their lives, in what they often perceive, despite the best efforts of their teachers, to be more of a prison than a place providing learning opportunities. Finally, in Chapter 10, we see how, though fortunately the situation is now better recognized and change may be on the way, the exclusion of young people in their teens from the workplace, means that, especially young people whose strengths are in practical skills rather than in academic subjects, are made to feel useless. At the same time, leisure facilities and creative opportunities for the young out of school are seriously inadequate.

It is, of course, good news for parents that around four out of five teenage children are neither unusually troubled nor troubling. Indeed, though at times they may be irritating, outrageous, and unpredictable, on balance their parents are likely to regard them as a source of pleasure and delight. All the same, the fact that as many as one in five young people in their teens has significant problems is a cause for concern. Further, though the evidence is, in fact, rather weak, there is a widespread impression and some support for the notion that some types of disruptive, especially violent behaviour and some ways of showing emotional upset, such as anorexia, do appear to be on the increase. Though those suffering from them are still in a minority, there are therefore widespread and possibly increasing numbers of young people with problems in the teen population.

11.2 The responsibility of the adult world for those in their teens

Even if there were no more problems now than existed in the past, the adult world should surely do what it can to improve matters. As we see in Chapter 2, in considering the enormously different lives those in their teens have lived in the past as well as what we can learn about the variety of ways in which the young have been treated in traditional societies, the adult world can, within very, very broad limits, fashion the teen years in the way it wants to. As we have seen, in some societies teens live in their families until they marry, in others they leave their parents' home at 13 or 14 to live with others of their age and never return home. In some societies, virginity is the rule until at least the mid-twenties, in others nearly all young people have had full sexual intercourse by the time they are 16 or 17 years of age. In all these societies, teens go through the same biological changes, experience the same increase in sex hormones as well as the same spurt in growth.

The physical changes that occur at this age do not therefore govern the sort of lives the young lead; that is decided by the rules of the society in which they live. If western adult society decided it wished to change the teen world, it could. In thinking what it might do, the adult world has, in general, taken the view that it will target the minority that is distressed and disruptive to see what it can do to prevent problems occurring or, much more commonly, what it can do to deal with them once they have reached serious proportions. But the fact is that the disturbed minority are only different from the rest of the adolescent population in the degree to which they are reacting to the powerless predicament in which young people find themselves. They are merely at one end of a continuum. If therefore adults wish to improve the situation of the minority, they will have to think about changing the situation of the whole adolescent population.

11.3 **How the adult world might sort out its own confusion about the teens**

The problems I have outlined do not all have precisely the same causes. But, as we have seen, there are certain common themes underlying all of them. In particular, unwillingness on the part of the adult world to consult and respect the views of young people, with underestimation of their potential competence and capacity to take responsibility for their own lives, seems to be pervasive.

In thinking about how to change the life of the teens, one starting point would be to try to sort out our confused ideas about those in their teens and about this phase of life called adolescence. It seems to be a confusing time for the young, but also makes the adult world behave in uncertain, confused ways. We say that those in their teens sometimes want to be treated like children and sometimes like grown ups. They don't know what they want. This is true, but perhaps we do not sufficiently allow for the fact that sometimes the adult world treats them like children and, at other times like fully developed adults. It is not just teenagers who do not know what they want from the teens; adults seem to have the same problem in reverse. So it is not surprising the teens are confused.

11.4 **Better protection for the pre-teen child: more adolescent empowerment**

As we move through the early years of the twenty-first century, perhaps both adult and adolescent confusion might be lessened if we started treating children as children, in need of a good deal of special protection, and adolescents as young, though inexperienced adults, competent to take decisions on their own behalf, and to live with the consequences of those decisions, much more often than we currently allow. The high rates of abuse of young children (nearly all of which takes place in the family), the younger and younger ages at which children are inappropriately sexualized (long before they have reached sexual maturity), the younger ages at which pre-teens are exposed to alcohol and illegal drugs, the judicial exposure of 10–14-year-olds to criminal proceedings on the grounds that they can take full responsibility for any criminal activity in which they have been involved—all these point to inadequate child protection.

In contrast, we allow a situation in which highly competent, physically mature young people, from the age of 14 and 15 years upwards, are infantilized in school, forbidden from sexual activity, and frustrated by their disempowered life situation to such a degree that they become depressed, sometimes suicidally so, or are tempted to engage in often seriously antisocial activity. We justify the constraints we put on teenagers with reference to their emotional immaturity, but as we have seen, when it suits the adult world, it is happy enough to give teenagers much greater responsibility.

Now, as we have seen, the young mature at very different rates. So, in an ideal world, the decision whether to allow young people to engage in adult activities would be taken on the basis of individual assessments of their level of competence. This is, after all, what happens in authoritative families all the time (see Chapter 3). It would also happen to a greater extent in schools if class sizes were smaller and teachers were able to escape the 'one size fits all' approach. Even at the present time, in one situation, the giving of information about conception and the means of conception, as well as consent to medical procedures, the use of the so-called Gillick principle (see page 240), the use of an approach based on competence rather than on chronological age, is sanctioned by case law.

But it is just not possible for every ruling on the age when young people are permitted to engage in adult activities to be undertaken on an individual basis. There just have to be statutory ages laid down for entitlement to a driving licence, to purchase of contraceptives in a chemist, to enter a public house, to buy alcoholic drinks, to leave school. Otherwise all these activities would require tests of competence before they were permitted.

On the other hand, the present situation, in which there are numerous different points in time at which the young become eligible to engage in these activities is confusing and inappropriate. Further, some of the restrictions at present in place, are largely ignored.

11.5 **The need to mark the beginning of adulthood**

One way of dealing with the confusion would be for the adult world to intro-duce a point in time, a particular age, when the young would be expected to take on most adult responsibilities and assume most adult rights. This is not such a radical change as it might seem. After all, there is no legal concept of adolescence; in law people are either adults or children and the distinction, apart from the application of the Gillick principle, is made by chronological age. (Incidentally the same situation holds in traditional societies. The well-known rites de passage all occur at one point in time, though not necessarily at one age. There is no society in which there is one ceremony to mark the transition from childhood to adolescence and another from adolescence to adulthood.) If our society wished to make a particular age a clear dividing point between childhood and adulthood, in deciding what this age should be, it would be necessary to take into account developmental processes, the potential competence of those in their teens, together with their needs for education and preparation for fully adult life.

Based on the information provided in earlier chapters, I would suggest that the age of 14 years would be the most appropriate point at which to mark the beginning of young adult life, and that this age should be recognized as such in our legal system and in our behaviour towards the young more generally. Let us see what this would mean in practice.

11.6 **The age of criminal responsibility**

If this suggestion were found acceptable, a first important step would be to raise the age of criminal responsibility to 14 years rather than, as at present, 10 years. Currently, in English and Welsh law, children over the age of 10 years are criminally responsible. In most other European countries, the age at which children can be prosecuted ranges from 13 to 18 years with a tendency to raise rather than lower the age. There has been widespread concern about the low age of criminal responsibility in England and Wales. (It is even lower, namely 8 years, in Scotland.) A working party of the organization, Justice, called in 1996 for urgent consideration of the issue. The working party pointed to evidence, already cited in this book, that the capacity for abstract thought rises up to 14 years, and that children's ability to feel guilt and shame and appreciate the long-term consequences of their actions increases with age up to this same point.

These changes in the age of criminal responsibility could be linked to changes in the courts in which children and young people were tried as well as to the system of custodial care. Though one would hope most young people charged would not be given custodial sentences, but would receive community sentences linked to rehabilitation programmes, if they were, there would be good reasons for these to be served in young adult institutions serving those aged 14 to say 25 years. A strong emphasis on rehabilitation would be required for the whole of this young adult population.

11.7 Community participation and the voting age

The voting age (currently 18 years) could be reduced, perhaps in the first instance to 16 years and then ultimately, though this is unlikely to happen for some time, to 14 years to bring it into line with the age of criminal responsibility and other changes to be proposed later in this chapter.

Such a change should not be seen in isolation, but as part of a strategy to engage young people in their teens in neighbourhood and community issues, as well as in local and national politics. As is well known, there is currently a sense of cynicism in the general population about the activities of politicians at all levels. This has led to a widespread feeling of detachment shown, for example, by the dropping turnout at local and national elections. The lack of interest is greatest in the young. In a sample of 580 twelve- to nineteen-year-olds, 64% said they had little or no interest in politics. Only 3% said they were interested a 'great deal'. Not surprisingly then, the proportion of young people casting their vote is lower than that of the rest of the population. For example, in the 2001 General Election only just over half the 18–24-year-olds voted compared to about two-thirds of the over 24s.

The young, like many in the adult population, are indeed unconvinced that politicians make a difference. Very few would consider joining a political party. Like the rest of the population, they distrust the integrity of politicians and see them as more interested in their own careers than in pursuing principled politics. This does not mean that they wish to see change achieved by violent means. Most decry the violence of the small minorities who attack the police at the meetings of world summit leaders. They support the democratic process. But they want to see this process tackling what they see as the real issues. How can they be persuaded that it is worthwhile for them to engage in the process themselves?

For the young are passionately interested in what *they* regard as the major issues of the day. It is simply that they have different priorities on their own political agenda. In the early months of 2003, thousands of teenagers took to the streets to protest against the war in Iraq. Young people have a strong, more enduring interest in environmental issues, especially if these are local ones. A MORI study carried out in 1999 reported that 82% of 11–16-year-olds thought they needed to understand global issues. Seventy percent were worried about world poverty. Environmental campaigns like those run by Greenpeace and Friends of the Earth attract large numbers of young people in their teens. Indeed the youth membership of Greenpeace rose from 80 000 in 1987 to 420 000 in 1995. Friends of the Earth reported a growth of 125 000 new young members over the same period. In contrast the Young Conservative membership in the early and mid-1990s was around 10 000.

Hugh Matthews and his colleagues have discussed the reasons for the lack of interest of young people in local and national politics. They point to the interest taken by the young in environmental issues as evidence that, given the right conditions, young people's energies could be positive forces for political change achieved through democratic processes. They suggest a number of reasons why the adult world fails to involve the young. Giving power to those in their teens is seen as threatening parental authority. Encouraging the young to become involved in local and national issues and to take some responsibility in decision-making is seen as 'stealing' their right to a childhood in which they should be free to grow without being troubled with the cares of the world. Neither of these objections has any serious validity. As we have seen in Chapter 4, children grow up better educated and more responsible precisely if they are encouraged to enter into debate with their parents. Childhood and the teen years are, in any case, not times of blissful ignorance and irresponsibility. Young people in today's world have their full share of worries and anxieties. Nor, as we have seen in Chapter 1, is there any basis for the view that young people in their teens do not have the intelligence or competence to understand political issues.

Instead of discouraging the young from political participation, the adult world should give attention to the ways in which, from early childhood, they can be engaged in making the world a better place for themselves and for others. Matthews and his colleagues suggest that this can be achieved by involving children of primary school age in local environmental management issues, such as recycling, wildlife surveys, and waste audits. By secondary school age, young people can begin to become involved in school councils, youth club committees, and young people's forums. Preparation for democratic participation in this way is far more likely to result in later interest in political issues than excluding the young from having any say in what goes on in the world in which they live. Carolyne Willow has also described a number of initiatives in which this is already happening.

All over the world there is now slow, but growing interest in finding ways to engage the interest of the young especially in local issues. This is especially noticeable in the development of Youth Councils. In mainland Europe, much progress has been made following the launch in 1992 of the Council of

Europe's 'European Charter on the participation of young people in municipal and regional life'. There are now many examples of active involvement of young people in political life. The Spanish Youth Council coordinates the activities of 70 organization, including 17 Regional Youth Councils. In France the growth of Conseils d'Enfants and de Jeunes has been rapid and there are now over 900 such Councils. Such Youth Councils can have a real impact, and, if they are to survive, they must have the capacity to make a difference. In Oslo, Norway, in 1999, I talked with leaders of the City's Youth Council, elected from the city population of under-18s, and asked if any of their deliberations really made a difference. I was told that, in the previous year the Youth Council had made an improvement in school buildings its priority. This had resulted in the City Council making a substantially greater increase to the relevant budget than had previously been planned.

In the UK progress has been slower, but, by the year 2000, there were already over 200 UK Youth Councils. Progress has been particularly rapid in Scotland, where there has been a development of a network of youth forums, and in Northern Ireland, where there is a strong network of Local Youth Councils. There is, as yet, little evidence that the deliberations of these Councils are taken seriously, though there is no doubt that some Chief Executives of Local Authorities are trying to ensure that the views of young people are taken into account in the provision of leisure facilities and in improvement of public transport, on which the young depend much more than do adults. There is also now an initiative to create a UK Youth Parliament, though it is debatable whether this is desirable in the light of the need to integrate young people into the world of responsible decision-making rather than segregate them from it. If the voting age were reduced, then there would be no need for a separate Youth Parliament. This would not be a new departure. The historian Hugh Thomas reports that in 1667, Christopher, the 14-year-old son of George Monck, opened a Commons debate.

To suggest the voting age for national elections should be reduced is not a new proposal. In 1996, a Report of the Gulbenkian Foundation recommended that the voting age should be lowered to 16 years with a corresponding lowering of the age at which young people can stand for election. Nor in 2002 is it a measure lacking current political support. It is official Liberal Democratic policy and is being actively discussed in the Labour Party's Young People's Forum. If the age of the franchise were reduced from 18 to 16 years, this would result in young people having the vote immediately after reaching compulsory school age. Participation in school affairs would be rapidly followed by the opportunity for involvement in local and national politics, to have the same amount of say in what goes on as the rest of the adult population.

After all, as we see in Chapter 10, an increasing number of under-18s are earning significant sums through e-commerce and many are now paying tax. The cry raised before the American Revolution 'No taxation without representation' now applies equally to this age group.

11.8 Reducing the age of consent to sexual intercourse to 14 years

Around one in five young people (slightly more males than females) have full sexual intercourse before the age of 16 years. The great majority of these have sex between the ages of 14 and 16 years. As we see in Chapter 6, the age of first intercourse dropped markedly in the 30 years from 1960 to 1990, but it is probably reasonably stable now. In the same chapter we also see that under-age girls have major difficulties in obtaining contraception. The teenage pregnancy rate is higher in the UK than in most other European countries.

Lowering the age of consent to 14 years for both boys and girls would mean that the roughly 120 000 girls aged 14–15 years in the UK who are having intercourse would no longer be breaking the law. The main argument against a change in the law is that it would send out the wrong sort of message, namely that it was quite acceptable for girls of 14 and 15 years to have sex. This does not seem to be the case in Austria and Italy, where the legal age of consent for girls is 14, or in Spain, where the age of consent is 12, but, where, in all three countries, the teenage pregnancy rate is lower than that in the UK, which has the highest in Europe. It should be added that there is no popular move towards lowering the age of consent, though, unsurprisingly, it is among young people themselves that there is the greatest support for this measure.

Since 1986, when the so-called Gillick case was heard, there has been much legal argument over the age at which girls should have the right to make decisions about medical investigations and treatment in opposition to their parents. Initially this argument was about contraceptive advice and whether this could be given by a doctor without the knowledge of the young person's parents. This has resulted in the development of common law, through the Gillick principle, that allows the doctor to take into account the understanding of the young person of the issues involved in making decisions about the need to involve parents. This principle is applied not just in decisions about contraception, but in all medical interventions. Interestingly it seems widely agreed, and this certainly seems sensible and in line with the views expressed elsewhere in this book, that the Gillick principle cannot be applied before the age of about 13 years, when it is reasonable to assume the child is not 'Gillick competent'. At any rate no case has been contested when the child has been below this age.

Michael Freeman has argued that the Gillick case established an important principle in law, namely that the capacity of the child, not the child's age, should be the important fact in deciding upon competence. While this is, of course, the way sensible parents behave in family life, and the way judges can now behave when asked to give attention to difficult medical cases, there would still seem to me to be clear advantages in deciding upon an age when the young can be assumed to be competent. Otherwise every young person would have to undergo an intelligence test before entering a pub or being given a provisional driving licence.

11.9 Raising the age of legally recognized part-time work to 14 years

Currently from the age of 13 years, children are legally allowed to work part-time, though only in certain jobs and subject to various conditions. In fact, as we see in Chapter 10, quite large numbers of children younger than this work on a part-time basis in the holidays and at weekends. Often they are helping out in family-owned shops or assisting the family in other ways. There are no good reasons why anyone should want to interfere with such informal arrangements, but 13 years seems rather a young age to enter legally regulated employment. Would it not be more sensible to bring the age up to 14 years, the age at which the 2002 Labour Government is proposing that secondary school students should enter work training more seriously than is the case now? Though this might be a premature suggestion, at some point attention should be given to reducing minimum wage regulations from 18 years as is the case now, at least down to 16 years.

11.10 Buying cigarettes and alcoholic drinks

In view of the current high rates of cigarette smoking and alcohol consumption in young people, it would be perverse to suggest that the ages when the young could buy cigarettes in a shop and alcohol in licensed premises should also be reduced to 14 years without suggesting other changes that would need to accompany such a change. In recent years, cigarette smoking in public places has gradually been banned. This is the case for most schools, theatres and cinemas, trains and planes, hospitals, and many restaurants. Many people find it offensive to have to inhale cigarette smoke wherever they are, and if the ban were extended to the street, this would mean that young people would only be able to smoke at home or, if they were allowed to enter them, licensed premises. (In fact, there has now been a small increase in the number of non-smoking pubs, so they too might eventually become no smoking areas.)

As young people already smoke at home just about as much as they want to and their parents can tolerate, reducing the age when they could buy cigarettes would not, in these circumstances, make any significant difference to their consumption. In fact, it might well reduce it significantly as some parents would ban smoking in their homes.

Similarly, reducing the age when the young could buy and consume alcohol in off-licenses and pubs to 14 years, though an unwise move in the absence of other changes, could well result in a drop in alcohol consumption in the young if it were accompanied by a general ban on drinking alcohol in public places, including the street. The young already drink at home as much as they wish. It is in the interests of landlords to prevent rowdy behaviour by young people in pubs if they want to keep their older customers. There is no reason to think that permitting 14–18-year-olds into pubs would make any significant difference, in itself, to the amount they drink. As I suggested in Chapter 7, it is the violence and other public displays of drunkenness, that accompany excessive drinking that are objectionable to the general public, and firmer measures to deal with these, no matter what the age of the offender, might well be followed by a drop in alcohol consumption in the young.

Incidentally, defining a single age when the young could purchase alcohol and consume it in licensed premises would make it easier to enforce the law in this respect. In contrast to many 16- and 17-year-olds, the great majority of 12- and 13-year-olds are obviously just not old enough to enter pubs and buy alcoholic drinks. It would also become easier to enforce a proof of age requirement in pubs and off-licences.

11.11 **Other changes helping to mark 14 years as the beginning of adulthood**

At the present time, there is considerable uncertainty about how best to provide beds for those in their teens who need in-patient medical or, much more commonly psychiatric care. Some Health Authorities provide adolescent beds for 12–19-year-olds, or 13–18-year-olds; others provide so-called young adult units for 16–25-year-olds, leaving the care of those under the age of 16 years as part of the children's service. If my suggestion that the age of 14 years should be seen as the beginning of young adulthood, then it would be logical to settle for the 14–25 pattern. Some people would be horrified at the thought of vulnerable 14-year-olds being on psychiatric units with mature 25-year-olds and that is an appropriate concern. However, the inadequate staff–patient ratios, frequency of staff changes, poor quality of staff training, and low staff morale on the units they are rightly concerned about make them unsatisfactory places for people of any age. If these units were really meeting the needs of disturbed 25-year-olds as many in fact do today, there would be no reason why they should not do the same for patients in earlier young adulthood.

11.12 **The need to retain some flexibility**

I am not, of course, suggesting that the age when a young person could obtain a driving licence should be cut down to 14 years. Indeed, it might well be raised to 18 years as it is in most other European countries. However, one advantage of lowering the age when the young could buy alcohol lawfully would be that it would mean there was more time for them to learn to control their alcohol intake before they started to drive. Better still would be the introduction of legalization to halve the level of alcohol in the blood at which it was an offence to drive from 80 micrograms per litre to 40 micrograms per litre, a move favoured anyway by most people concerned about the high rate of alcohol linked fatalities on our roads.

It would also be unwise to lower the age, currently 18 years, when the state relinquishes responsibility for children in public care. So many of such children are emotionally immature and traumatized; they need continued protection and support at least up to the age of 18 years, and often beyond.

11.13 **Music, films, and books: where lines are drawn**

Increasingly over the last 30 years popular music, initially aimed at the mid to late teens has been targeted at a wider and wider age span, spreading backwards to the tweens and forwards to the student population in their twenties. The de-emphasis of the lyric and the significance of the beat mean that appreciation does not require any particular level of intellectual capacity. Insofar as the contents of words of lyrics do have significance, they now have relevance to the whole age range. In the 1950s and 1960s when a popular lyric went 'They tried to tell us we're too young/Too young to really be in love/They say that love's a word/A word we've only heard/We can't begin to know the meaning of' it was those aged nineteen and twenty who probably identified most with the lyric's sentiment. Now if the song were revived (an improbable event!), it would probably be the 12- and 13-year-olds who would identify most strongly. Is this really appropriate?

At the beginning of the twenty-first century, much popular culture is aimed not only at the whole tween and teen population, but at the whole range of adults, from young to old, as well. The appeal of the magical world of Harry Potter, and the fantasies of J.R. Tolkien and Philip Pullman crosses generational boundaries. This is no new phenomenon. Robinson Crusoe,

Gulliver's Travels, Little Women, and indeed the novels of Charles Dickens were read by all, from the teens to the elderly, but not, except very occasionally, by the pre-teens.

In books only aimed at the literate proportion of the population of young people who read books for pleasure, there is recognition of the difference between the younger reader in the 9–13 age group and the older teen reader, a difference well illustrated in the way such books are displayed in bookshops. Once it is possible to take account of the greater capacity of the post-thirteen age group, themes become more adult, and the complexity of relationships more accurately and profoundly described.

I suggested in Chapter 5 that the categories used by the British Board of Film Classification (BBFC) allowed too much violence to be shown at the '12' and '15' levels. In line with the other proposals in this chapter, it might be more logical to think of a simple '13–' and '14+' classification, abolishing the '12' and '18' categories. Sadly, the horrific levels of violence permitted at '18' rule this out. If we cannot protect vulnerable older people from images we can at least try, even if ineffectively, to protect those up to the age of 15 years.

11.14 A ceremony to mark the beginning of adulthood

I suggested in Chapter 9 that 14 years, or the beginning of Key Stage 4, the point at which young people begin preparation for public examinations, might be marked by some ceremony to which parents would be invited towards the beginning of that school year. The school might then recognize the new phase of life young people had entered with the granting of new rights and the taking on of new responsibilities that I proposed in that chapter. Of course, if reaching the age of 14 years also marked the assumption of legal rights and responsibilities and a change in the way the world outside school regarded young adults, this ceremony would take on much added significance.

11.15 Better preparation and protection for children under the age of 14 years

Establishing the age of 14 years as the point at which entry to most adult activities, would bring with it the need to provide better preparation for these activities before that age. But establishing this age as the formal beginning of young adulthood would make it easier for parents, teachers, and under-14-year-olds themselves to view those aged ten to thirteen as still definitely children, not the highly sexualized mini-adults as so many 10–13-year-olds are today. These years will, all the same, be especially crucial, as they are today in preparation for the rights and responsibilities of adulthood.

As we see in Chapter 3, preparation for adult life really begins in the family in the very early years of a child's life. I described in that chapter the evidence that certain types of parenting, already widely practiced, have been shown to be effective in producing emotionally well-balanced young people, achieving as well in their studies and in their later careers as their potential allowed. Such parenting practices have been shown to have this positive effect in all social classes and in all societies in which parenting has been studied. They involve treating children as individuals from their earliest days, respecting and taking account of the way they respond, listening carefully to them once they begin to talk, and involving them in decision-making, though by no means necessarily giving in to their wishes as soon as this is possible.

In the maintenance of discipline, it involves an emphasis on clear guidance on boundaries between what is and is not permitted, consistency in the application of rules, and an emphasis on rewards for good behaviour rather than punishment for bad. Above all, it requires parents to care lovingly for their children and to remain dependable supports throughout their childhood. It does not require parents to be perfect, but it does ask them to be 'good enough'.

Such parenting, moving gradually from an authoritative to a democratic mode as the child gets older, contrasts with authoritarian, punitive parenting practices, as well as with over-permissive, over-indulgent, and negligent parenting.

11.16 **Parent education**

As I indicated in Chapter 3, most parents manage to provide the type of optimum parenting I have described without any additional help. But there must be rather few who do not find it helpful at times to talk to relatives and friends, even occasionally taking professional advice, when they run into difficulties with their children, or are uncertain how to approach the next phase of their children's lives.

In the earlier chapter, I described some of the mainly voluntary services that exist in the UK to help parents and the young themselves when they run into difficulties. Some parent education programmes have now been shown to be effective in helping parents of young children to change their practices so that their children have a better chance of experiencing fewer problems in the future. Programmes for parents of teenage children are less well established, but some such programmes do exist that are well appreciated by parents even if they have not been demonstrated to be effective in changing behaviour. They should be more generally available.

Any discussion of parent education must raise questions about the relevance of such education for parents in families living in socially deprived circumstances, overcrowded, and short of money. Parents living in such circumstances can be helped by educational programmes, but it is important that these are relevant to their social situations. Further, governments need to recognize that the reduction of income inequalities and increase in the stock of decent housing stock would go a long way to improve the lives of families with teenage children and enable parents in such families to manage their children's difficulties more effectively.

11.17 **Discouragement of premature sexualization**

Encouraging sexual awareness and sexually provocative behaviour increases the risk that children will experience sexual feelings and become entangled in sexual relationships they just cannot handle. First sexual experiences are likely to involve a confused mixture of anticipation, excitement, intense pleasure, dread of loss, jealousy, and uncertainty about the future at whatever age they occur. It is unfair, even cruel to expect children to be able to cope with these intense emotions until they have developed some degree of emotional maturity. This is not likely to occur until their mid-teens.

Of course there is no clear dividing line for parents between dressing their children or encouraging them to dress attractively and dressing or encouraging them to dress in a sexually provocative manner. The line between charming and seductive manners is similarly blurred. But most parents in social situations with other adults are well aware when they themselves, by the way they dress or behave, are out to sexually provoke or to seduce and when they merely wish to be pleasing and good company. They can and indeed most do help their children develop similar social skills.

The fashion business and the magazines for those in their early teens do not make this task any easier for parents. The Lolita look, in whatever contemporary fashionable form it takes, is good for sales. Because of the blurred line between attractive and sexually provocative appearance it is only possible to ban the most excessively inappropriate images of sexually immature children. But it is important for responsible editors and journalists to think seriously about the publication of such images and for teachers in Personal, Social Health Education (PSHE) classes to continue to point to their inappropriateness and possible dangers. A society that allows publication of such images without criticism cannot escape responsibility for some of the paedophilic activity that so preoccupies and angers it.

In most western societies, children tend to mix in same-sex groups in the years before puberty. Though this occurs in many societies, there is nothing inevitably biological about it. It happens at least partly because parents bring boys and girls up differently from an early age. The encouragement of mixed-sex, non-sexual friendships from an early age could help to prevent the sort of stereotyping that makes it seem as though the two sexes live on different planets. Then by the time of puberty, boys and girls would not view each other as members of alien species, but as human beings with similar needs. The attitudes of boys and girls to sexual relationships would still doubtless be somewhat different, but there would be more common ground in terms of their social skills, past experiences, and present interests. It would be particularly helpful in early boy–girl sexual relationships if, during childhood, both sexes had learned ways of sorting out differences and disagreements in a non-violent manner, boys without resorting to physical force and girls without mockery and humiliation. Men may be from Mars and women from Venus, but they need to be able to get on together on this planet Earth, and childhood is a good time to start making this happen.

11.18 **Preparation for adulthood in the school curriculum**

In most of the previous chapters in this book, I have put emphasis on the need to take seriously the PSHE in the school curriculum and to make it not just a desirable, but a compulsory part of the syllabus. A sound framework to enable teachers to deliver this subject exists in the form of guidance for PSHE published by the Department for Education and Skills. During Key Stage 3, generally completed by around the age of 14 years, students are expected to learn how to develop confidence and responsibility, and make the most of their abilities. Under this heading, it is recommended they should be taught:

- How to recognize how others see them, and be able to give and receive constructive feedback and praise.
- Recognize the stages of emotions associated with loss and change caused by death, divorce, separation, and new family members ...
- The influences on how we spend or save money and how to become competent at managing personal money.

Under the heading of developing a healthy, safer lifestyle, they should learn:

- To recognize the physical and emotional changes that take place at puberty ...
- Basic facts and laws, including school rules, about alcohol and tobacco, illegal substances, and the risks of misusing prescribed drugs.

+ In the context of relationships, about human reproduction, contraception, sexually transmitted infections, HIV, and high-risk behaviours including early sexual activity.

Similarly invaluable curricular guidance is provided under the headings of 'Developing good relationships and respecting the differences between people' and 'Breadth of opportunities', which give students the experience of working together with others on projects and finding information and advice about high-risk activities for themselves.

Excellent guidance for teachers to help the under 14s prepare for adulthood therefore exists. The catch is that, at the time of writing in 2002, there is very little teacher training in this subject, many teachers find it difficult to teach without such training, and therefore, not surprisingly, the subject is not popular with them. As I indicated in Chapter 9, it is not an obligatory part of the National Curriculum. Consequently, although it is at least as valuable a part of the school curriculum as most, if not all of the subjects that are compulsorily included, it is often given much less skilled and committed attention than it deserves.

11.18.1 Empowerment in family life

If we think of the age of 14 years as the time when a young person has reached young adult status, and is not just in the middle of some treacherous, poorly defined no man's land called adolescence, what, if anything, would this mean for family life?

When a group of adults live together in the same household, they do not all act independently of each other. They take account of each other's needs and wishes. The more experienced give advice and support to the less experienced. Supportive parents of young people of this age would inevitably find themselves in this role, but would not have the final say in what their children did. Their children would not wish to upset them, but, as is the case now, might take decisions of which it was clear their parents disapproved.

Does this mean that 14- and 15-year-olds would be able to choose to come in at night at whatever time they wanted? Yes, they would. But obviously their parents would have the right to tell them they would prefer them to come home by say 10 or 11 pm. If they disturbed other members of the family when they came in, there would be a need for the sort of negotiation that goes on between adults to sort matters out. If they got into trouble with the police while they were out, they would be fully responsible for their actions, and their parents could not be held to account for behaviour over which they had no control. That is what adulthood is about. Would they be able to decide not to do homework they were set? Yes, they would, but if their examination results were poor, they would have only themselves and not their parents to blame. Again, that is what adulthood is about.

Although this may seem to suggest there should be a rather radical change in the power balance between parents and their children, in practice, the situation would not be very different from that which exists in most families at the present time. In general, if young people in their mid-teens wish to act in a particular way, there is very little their parents can do to stop them. Parents can reduce or stop pocket money now, in the same way that any adults making voluntary payments to other adults can cease to do so if they wish. That would not change. In theory, parents can 'ground' their teenage children. But in fact this can only really occur if their children agree to it. That too would not change. Parents could ask their children to tell them where they were going in the evening and to provide a contact telephone number, in the same way as any adults living in the same household would be entitled to ask of each other.

Would teenage children respect their parents less? That is a possibility, but it is more likely that parents would be accorded more rather than less respect when their children experienced for themselves the difficulties that come with taking full responsibility for oneself. What would be different would be the loss of the fiction that parents can actually control young people of this age, and that governments and other authorities are therefore right to blame them when their children behave badly. Of course, parents would continue to blame themselves when things did not work out well for their teenage children; so do parents of 20- and 30-year-olds.

11.18.2 **Empowerment in school**

In Chapter 9 I pointed to a number of ways in which some schools were now empowering students at secondary level. They included:

- Giving students regular opportunities to comment on the performance of their teachers in the same way that teachers provide feedback to students.
- Involving students in the selection of teaching staff.
- Giving students more say in the choice of their own courses of study.
- Making the curriculum more relevant to the needs of all students, by making PSHE a statutory subject.
- Using more interactive methods in the classroom.
- Giving students more opportunity to teach others, and thus to consolidate their knowledge.
- Limiting the number of examinations students take and providing more opportunities for assessing performance by using criteria developed in consultation with the student.

- Involving students in the organization of their schools to a greater degree, for example in the prevention of bullying, in active participation in School Councils, and by giving them more opportunities to carry out tasks in school as part of their work experience.

- Recognizing that 'turning round' schools failing because they were in 'challenging circumstances' involved amongst, of course, many other measures, empowering those students who really wanted to see the school as a learning environment.

- Recognizing the diversity of student needs by allowing variation in the pace of learning and examination taking as well as the subjects for study, so that unusually fast learners, those who found academic study difficult and those who were more talented in practical subjects could all feel their needs were being met and they were performing well.

- Using information technology much more widely in order to individualize learning.

- Ensuring school equipment and buildings were all maintained at a high level, so that both students and staff could feel proud of their environment and have confirmation that the community valued their work.

11.19 Joining up 14+ young adults to the rest of the adult world

Removing anomalies in the law that affect the teens, and preparing the young better for the adult world, will not, in themselves affect the degree to which those of this age group are separated from the rest of the human race. Such separation is one of the causes of the stigmatization of those in their teens that I described in the first chapter. Many of the myths about the teenage years occur because of the fact that most of the adult world, apart from their parents and secondary school teachers, does not have much contact with them. Further, it is to the disadvantage of those in their teens that their separation from the adult world (other than parents and teachers) means they cannot benefit from contact with those who have more experience than they do. The teens need joining up.

The natural response to this suggestion is that teenagers do not want to be joined up. Their main concern is to be like other teenagers, especially those who are high status because they are good-looking, popular, good fun, not too hard working or clever and, if they are boys, successfully athletic. Peer pressure is usually not an issue. If those with high status around them are behaving in a particular way, that is the way they will want to behave; they do not need to be pressured to do so. But the assumption that 'hanging out with the group' is their *only* interest is a symptom of the dismissive attitude of the adult world to those in their teens. Most are happy to spend time in other ways.

In fact, there is much that can be done both in family life, at school, and in the neighbourhood not just to help the teens maintain contact with the adult world, but actually to strengthen such contact to the benefit of both teenagers and older people. The assumption that all activities set up by adults for young people are rejected by them is false. For example, many sports clubs and music groups are found very acceptable by those in their teens. Many families have found it possible to keep their teenage children engaged, even if they do prefer, as most will, to go out with their friends.

11.20 Joining up the teens through family life

What can family members, especially parents but also, if they are around, older brothers and sisters do to retain contact with their teenagers? First, they can avoid pretending to be of teen age themselves. They can continue to provide a home that is welcoming and interested in them, not just food and a bed. At least as importantly they can give moral support and advice when it is requested, when times are tough and depressing for their children. They can offer activities that bring together family members of different generations, such as family get-togethers at Christmas, birthdays, and other celebrations, with teenagers included no matter how outlandish they may look. The young often need little persuasion to go on family holidays if they are being paid for and the venue is attractive, though only the better off are likely to be able to afford this means of keeping the family together. Parents can provide opportunities for their teenage children to talk with grandparents, aunts and uncles, and old family friends, who may be easier for them to relate to than parents. Participating together in a sporting activity or family membership of a health club often strengthens contact between parents and their teenage children. Family friends and relatives can provide careers advice and help in finding part-time work. In fact, as Virginia Morrow and Martin Richards have found, more young people find their first job through a contact with a member of the family or a friend than through career guidance at school.

11.21 Joining up the teens in schools and colleges of further education

For secondary age students, most contact with the adult world outside the family is with teachers. Most adults will remember one or more teachers who had an influence on them while they were at school through opportunities outside the classroom, perhaps on school journeys or, as far as boys are concerned, on coach trips visiting other schools to play away fixtures. Because teachers are busy and because, after all, they represent a rather narrow stratum of society, increasingly schools and the government are looking for ways to make contacts with other sections of the adult world.

Connexions, a support service for young people, was set up in the year 2000, and after two years was in full-scale operation in 26 areas of the UK, with a plan to cover the whole country after another two years. The aim is to extend the role of the Careers service to help young people who are in difficulties, often because they come from disadvantaged backgrounds, to tackle barriers to learning, and give them advice on career and learning goals. Just how successful this scheme will be is not known.

The UK Home Office and Department for Education and Skills is also supporting a number of mentoring schemes. Mentoring has been defined as a process whereby 'an older, more experienced person takes a younger person under his/her wing, freely offering advice, support, and encouragement. The mentor becomes, among other things, a role model who inspires the younger person' (North London College). Increasingly, banks, accountancy, and law firms as well as manufacturing businesses are seconding younger members of their staff to undertake mentoring tasks in secondary schools on a half-day a week or one day a fortnight basis. With the right sort of personality, ability to listen, relate, and be supportive, together with appropriate training, many mentors have proved their value in helping secondary school students overcome barriers to learning and plan their lives more effectively.

The increasing emphasis on lifelong learning provides other possibilities for the young to be joined up to the adult world. Although this seems to happen rather rarely, there could be more opportunities made for older people who wish to study subjects that are taught to 16–19-year-olds in Colleges of Further Education to do so in the same classroom. In some places retired people who wish to learn computer skills are being taught by secondary school students, who consolidate their own knowledge in this way.

11.22 **Joining up the teens in the community**

Earlier in this chapter I described a number of ways in which young people in their teens are involved and could certainly be more involved in neighbourhood projects, especially in planning and carrying out improvements to the environment. In Chapter 10 I described ways in which more opportunities could be made for young people of this age not just to gain 'work experience', valuable though this is, but also to have proper jobs with a reasonable wage. All links with the world of work inevitably bring young people into contact with older, more experienced people. In the same chapter, I discuss how the young can be joined up to the adult world in leisure activities.

If more adults had contact with those in their teens, the young would benefit from the wisdom and experience of older people and they in turn would be less likely to cling to the misconceptions they hold about the young. That, surely, cannot do anything but good.

Such an approach would require us to rethink the purpose of adolescence or the teen years. At the present time, the adult world seems to think of the teen years like a shuttle bus at an airport. Picked up at one terminal called Childhood, the young are conveyed on a shuttle call Adolescence, and deposited at a second terminal called Adulthood. This view of adolescence as an in-between stage is unhelpful. Adolescence need not just be a preparation for adulthood but the beginning of adult life. Competent 14–19 year olds need the respect accorded to young adults, not the condescension displayed to those who are still virtually children.

Further Reading

There is an enormous amount of literature on the topics covered in this book. For each chapter, I have listed a number of key references. The number of the page in which information provided by the reference is relevant is given in brackets after it.

Introduction

Guides for Parents of Teenagers

Aidan Macfarlane and Ann McPherson (2000) *Teenagers.* Warner Books, London.
Kate Figes (2002) *The terrible teens.* Viking, London.

Textbooks on Adolescence

Michael Jaffe (1998) *Adolescence.* John Wiley, Chichester.
John Coleman and Leo Hendry (1999) *The nature of adolescence.* Routledge, London.

Chapter 1

Edward Albee Finding the Sun. Dramatists Play Service, Inc. (5)
James Tanner (1990) *Fetus into man.* Harvard University Press, Cambridge, Mass. (9)
Daniel Offer and Kimberley Schonert-Reichl (1992) Debunking the myths of adolescence: findings from recent research. *Journal of the American Academy of Child and Adolescent Psychiatry,* **31**, 1003–14. (12)
Criminal Statistics, England and Wales 2001. Research, Development and Statistics Directorate and National Statistics, 2002. (12)
Office of National Statistics (1998) *Abortion Statistics.* Stationery Office, London. (13)
Weithorn, L.A. and Campbell, S.B. (1982) The competency of children to make informed treatment decisions. *Child Development,* **53**, 1589–98. (13)
Robert Sternberg (1988) *The triarchic mind.* Viking, New York. (15)
Jeffrey Jensen Arnett (2000) Emerging adulthood. *American Psychologist,* **55**, 469–81. (15)
Jay Giedd (1999) Brain development. IX Human brain growth. *American Journal of Psychiatry,* **156**, 4. (16)
Barbara Rausch (2003) Why are they so weird? What's really going on in a teenager's brain? Bloomsbury, London. (16)
Daniel Keating (1990) Adolescent Thinking. In Shirley Feldman and Glen Elliott (Eds) *At the threshold: The developing adolescent.* Harvard University Press, Cambridge, Mass. (17)
Erik Eriksen (1968) *Identity, youth and crisis.* W. W. Norton, New York. (17–18)
Stanovitch, K., West, R., Harrison, M. (1995) Knowledge, growth and maintenance across the life span. *Developmental Psychology,* **31**, 811–26. (13–17)
Mike Males (1996) *The Scapegoat Generation.* Common Courage Press, Monroe, Maine. (23)

James Cote and Anton Allaher (1994) *Generation on hold. Coming of age in the twentieth century.* New York University Press, New York. (24)

Chapter 2

Ilana Krausman Ben-Amos (1994) *Adolescence and youth in early modern England.* Yale University Press, London. (25–27)

John Burrow (1986) *The ages of man: A study in mediaeval writing and thought.* Oxford University Press, Oxford. (25–27)

John and Virginia Demos (1969) Adolescence in historical perspective. *Journal of Marriage and the Family,* **31,** 623–8. (25–27)

John Gillis (1974) *Youth and history: Tradition and change in European Age relations: 1770 to the present.* Academic Press, New York. (28–30)

Kett, S. (1977) *Rites of passage: Adolescence in America, 1790 to the present.* Basic Books, New York. (28–30)

Thomas Hine (1999) *The rise and fall of the American teenager.* Avon, New York.

Johann Wolfgang von Goethe (1989) *The sorrows of young Werther.* Penguin Classics, London. (28)

Stanley Hall, G. (1904) *Adolescence.* Appleton, New York. (28)

Peter Blos (1970) *The young adolescent.* Collier-Macmillan, London. (29)

Anna Freud (1952) Adolescence. *Psychoanalytic Study of the Child,* **13,** 255–278. (29)

Donald Winnicott (1971) Adolescence: struggling through the doldrums. *Adolescent Psychiatry,* **1,** 40–41. (29)

John Springhall (1986) *Coming of age: Adolescence in Britain: 1860–1960.* (30–35)

Robert Roberts (1973) *The Classic Slum.* Penguin Books, London. (31)

James McPherson (1988) *Battle cry of freedom: The American Civil War.* Oxford University Press, Oxford. (33)

Oserby, W. (1998) *Youth in Britain since 1945.* Blackwells, Oxford. (35–38)

Mark Abrams (1961) *The teenage consumer.* London Press Exchange, London. (35)

Andy Furlong and Fred Cartmel (1997) *Young people and social change.* Open University Press, Buckingham. (36)

Margaret Mead (1943) *Coming of age in Samoa.* Penguin Books, Harmondsworth. (38)

Alice Schlegel and Herbert Barry (1991) *Adolescence: An anthropological enquiry.* Free Press, New York. (39)

Sami Timimi (1985) Adolescence in immigrant Arab families. *Psychotherapy,* **32,** 141–9. (40)

Klaus Riegel (1972) Influence of economic and political ideologies on the development of developmental psychology. *Psychological Bulletin,* **78,** 129–41. (40–41)

Robert Enright and others (1987) Do economic conditions influence how theorists see adolescence? *Journal of Youth and Adolescence,* **16,** 541–60. (41)

Allison James and Alan Prout (1990) *Constructing and reconstructing childhood.* Falmer Press, London. (42)

Patrice Huerre and Colleagues (1997) *L'Adolescence n'existe Pas.* Odile Jacob, Paris. (42–43)

Chapter 3

Howard Melzer, Robert Goodman, and colleagues (2000) *The Mental Health of Children and Adolescents in Great Britain.* The Stationery Office, London. (46)

Nick Rand (2002) *Teenagers' lives in the twenty first century.* Report Commissioned by B SkyB. Future Foundation, London. (47)

Judith Rich Harris (1998) *The nurture assumption.* Bloomsbury, London. (48)

Diana Baumrind (1968) Authoritarian vs authoritative parental control. *Adolescence*, **3**, 255–272. (49)

ChildLine (1998) *Annual Report.* ChildLine, London. (49)

Farber, E.D. and Joseph, J. (1985) The maltreated adolescent: patterns of physical abuse. *Child Abuse and Neglect*, **9**, 201–6. (50)

NSPCC (1999) *The abuse of adolescents within the family.* NSPCC, London. (50)

Noom, M.J. and colleagues (1999) Autonomy, attachment and psychological adjustment during adolescence: a double-edged sword? *Journal of Adolescence*, **22**, 771–83. (57)

Lindsay Chase-Lansdale and colleagues (1994) A psychological perspective on the development of caring in children and youth. *Journal of Adolescence*, **18**, 515–556. (57)

Michael Willmott (2000) *Complicated lives.* Report commissioned by Abbey National. Future Foundation, London. (59)

Saul Becker and colleagues (1998) *Young carers and their families.* Blackwells, Oxford. (60)

Ian Butler and others (2002) Children's Involvement in their parent's divorce. *Children and Society*, **16**, 89–102. (63)

Chapter 4

Ian Goodyer (2001) *The depressed child and adolescent.* (2 ed). Cambridge University Press, Cambridge. (69–76)

Howard Melzer, Robert Goodman, and colleagues (2000) *The mental health of children and adolescents in Great Britain.* The Stationery Office, London. (71)

Peter Hoare and colleagues (1993) The modification and standardisation of the Harter Self-Esteem Questionnaire with Scottish schoolchildren. *European Child and Adolescent Psychiatry*, **2**, 19–33. (71–2)

Elizabeth Monck and Colleagues (1994) Adolescent girls: Self reported mood disturbance in a community population. *British Journal of Psychiatry* **165**, 760–9. (72–73)

Michael McLure, G. (2000) Changes in suicide rate in England and Wales, 1960–1997. *British Journal of Psychiatry*, **176**, 64–7. (74)

Christy Miller Buchanan and colleagues (1992) Are adolescents victims of raging hormones: evidence for activational effects of hormones on moods and behavior at adolescence. *Psychological Bulletin*, **111**, 62–107. (75)

Morton Seligman (1990) *Helplessness: On depression, development and death.* Freeman, San Francisco. (76)

Gael Lindenfield (2001) *Confident teens.* Thorsons, London. (82)

Philip Graham and Carol Hughes (2004) *So young, so sad, so listen.* Gaskell Press, London. (85)

Chapter 5

Youth Justice Board (2002) *Mori 2002 Youth Survey.* Youth Justice Board for England and Wales, London. (91)

Laurence Steinberg (1986) The vicissitudes of autonomy in early adolescence. *Child Development*, **57**, 841–51. (93)

Ungar, M.T. (2000) The myth of peer pressure. *Adolescence,* **35,** 167–180. (94)

Richard Jessor (Ed) (1998) *New perspectives on adolescent risk behavior.* Cambridge University Press, Cambridge. (94)

Judith Rich Harris (1998) *The nurture assumption.* Bloomsbury, London. (94)

Ruth Beyth-Marom and others (1993) Perceived consequences of risky behaviour: adults and adolescents. *Developmental Psychology,* **29,** 549. (95)

Claire Flood-Page and colleagues (2000) *Youth crime: Findings from the 1998/99 survey.* Home Office, London. (97)

Terrie Moffitt (1993) Adolescence limited and life course persistent antisocial behaviour: a developmental taxonomy. *Psychological Taxonomy,* **100,** 674–701. (98)

Terrie Moffitt and others (2001) *Sex differences in antisocial behaviour.* Cambridge University Press, Cambridge. (103)

Matt Sanders and colleagues (1996) *Every parent's survival guide (videotape and booklet).* Families International, Brisbane, Australia. (105)

Caroline Webster-Stratton (1998) Training for parents of young children with conduct problems: contents, methods and therapeutic processes. *Handbook of Parent Training,* 98–152. (105)

Stephen Scott and Kathy Sylva (1997) *Enabling parents: supporting specific parenting skills with a community programme.* Department of Health, London. (105)

Scott Henggeler and colleagues (2002) *Serious emotional disturbances in children and adolescents: Multisystemic therapy.* Guilford Press, London. (106)

British Board of Film Classification (2000) *Sense and sensibilities.* Public Opinion and the BBFC Guidelines. British Board of Film Classification, London. (114)

Chapter 6

James Tanner (1990) *Fetus into Man.* Cambridge University Press, Cambridge. (121–2)

Russell Viner (2002) Is puberty getting earlier in girls? *Archives of Disease in Childhood,* **84,** 8. (123)

Kaye Wellings and colleagues (1994) *Sexual behaviour in Britain.* Penguin Books, London. (124–127)

Martin Richards (1996) The childhood environment and the development of sexuality. In Henry C. and Ulijaszele S. (eds) *Long term consequences of early environment.* Cambridge University Press, Cambridge. (126)

Udry, J. and Billy, J. (1987) Initiation of coitus in early adolescence. *American Review of Sociology,* **52,** 841–55. (126)

Office of National Statistics (1998) *Abortion Statistics.* Stationery Office, London. (127)

Social Exclusion Unit (1999) *Teenage pregnancy.* HMSO, London. (128)

Holland, J. and colleagues (1991) *Pressured pleasure: Young women and the negotiation of sexual boundaries.* Tufnell Press, London. (129)

Mellanby, A.R. and colleagues (1995) School sex education: an experimental programme with educational and medical benefit. *BMJ,* **311,** 414–7. (129, 143)

Susan Moore and Deborah Rosenthal (1993) *Sexuality in adolescence.* Routledge and Kegan Paul, London. (129)

Danny Wight and colleagues (2000) Extent of regretted sexual intercourse among young teenagers in Scotland: a cross sectional survey. *BMJ,* **320,** 1243–4. (131)

Brook Advisory Centres (1998) *What people want from sex advice services.* Brook Advisory Centres, London. (139–147)

Roger Ingham (1998) Exploring interactional competence: Comparative data from the United Kingdom and the Netherlands on Young People's Sexual Development. Paper presented at 24th meeting of the International Academy of Sex Research, Sirmione, Italy 3–6 June 1998. (141)

Chapter 7

Ungar, M.T. (2000) The myth of peer pressure. *Adolescence,* **35,** 167–180. (152)

Royal College of Physicians (1995) *Alcohol and the young.* Report of a joint committee of the British Paediatric Association and Royal College of Physicians. Royal College of Physicians, London. (153)

Home Office Standing Committee on Crime Prevention (1987) *Young people and alcohol.* Report of a working group. Home Office, London. (153)

John Balding (2002) *Young people in 2001.* Schools Health Education Unit, Exeter. (153)

John Coleman and June Schofield (2003) Key data on adolescence. Trust for the study of Adolescence. TSA Publishing, Brighton. (154, 165)

The 1999 ESPAD Report—*The European school survey report on alcohol and other drugs.* Alcohol and Health Research Centre, Greenbank Drive, Edinburgh, Scotland EH10 5SB. (154)

Alcohol Concern (2000) *Britain's ruin.* Meeting Government Objectives via a National Alcohol Strategy, Alcohol Concern, London. (157)

Michael Windle (1999) *Alcohol use among adolescents.* Sage Publications, London. (158)

Griffiths Edwards, *et al.* (1994) *Alcohol policy and the public good.* Oxford Medical Publications, Oxford. (160)

Royal College of Psychiatrists (2000) *Drugs, dilemmas and choices.* Gaskell Press, London. (162, 165, 171)

Health Education Authority (1998) *A parent's guide to drugs and alcohol.* Health Education Authority, London. (162)

Chapter 8

Alissa Quart (2003) Branded: The Buying and Selling of Teenagers. Arrow, London. (173)

John Reilly and others (1999) Epidemic of obesity in UK children. *Lancet,* **354,** 1874. (174)

The Food Commission (2001) *Children's Nutrition Action Plan.* The Food Commission, 94, White Lion Street, London, N1. (175)

Hill, A. and colleagues (1992) Eating in the adult world. The rise in dieting during childhood and adolescence. *British Journal of Clinical Psychology,* **31,** 95–105. (176)

Arthur Crisp (1980) *Let me be.* Academic Press, London. (181)

Anne Becker and others (2002) Eating behaviours and attitudes following prolonged exposure to television among ethnic Fijian adolescent girls. *British Journal of Psychiatry,* **180,** 509. (184)

Nasser, M. (1997) *Culture and weight consciousness.* Brunner-Routledge, London. (184)

Steven Gortmaker and others (1999) Reducing obesity via a school based interdisciplinary intervention among youth: Planet Health. *Archives of Pediatric and Adolescent Medicine,* **153,** 409–18. (185)

Leonard Epstein and others (2000) Decreasing sedentary behaviors in treating pediatric obesity. *Archives of Pediatric and Adolescent Medicine*, **154**, 220. (185)

Chapter 9

Stephens, W. B. (1998) *Education in Britain. 1750–1914.* Macmillan, Basingstoke. (189)

Robert Roberts (1973) *The classic slum.* Penguin Books, London. (191)

Jacki Gordon and Gillian Grant (1997) *How we feel: An insight into the emotional world of teenagers.* Jessica Kingsley, London. (191)

Laurie Lee (1959) *Cider with Rosie.* Penguin Books, London. (191)

Michael Barber (1996) *The learning game.* Victor Gollancz, London. (193)

Lynne Davies (1999) *School Councils and Pupil Exclusion.* Schools Council, London. (196, 206)

Independent, 4 July, 2002. A Matter of Taste for Swedish Teachers. (196)

Article by Hilary Wilce, Guardian, 6, March, 2003. (196)

Department for Education and Employment (2001) *Building for success: a consultation document.* DfEE, London. (199)

John Gray and colleagues (1983) *Reconstructions of secondary education.* Routledge and Kegan Paul, London. (199)

Katherine Weare (2000) *Promoting mental, emotional and social health: a whole school approach.* Routledge, London. (199)

Joan Ruddock and colleagues (1996) *School improvement: what can pupils tell us?* David Fulton, London. (200)

Department for Education and Employment (1998) *Education for Citizenship and the Teaching of Democracy in Schools.* Department for Education and Employment, London. (202)

Dan Olweus (1993) *Bullying at school: What we know and what we can do.* Blackwell, Oxford. (205)

Martin Johnson (1999) *Failing school, failing city.* Charlbury, Jon Carpenter. (207)

Chapter 10

Jacki Gordon and Gillian Grant (1997) *How we feel: An insight into the emotional world of teenagers.* Jessica Kingsley, London. (213)

Anita Franklin and Nicola Madge (2000) *Young Lewisham: Consumer views on services for young people.* NCB, London. (213)

Tim Gill (2002) National Children's Play Council. *Personal Communication.* (214)

ChildWise (2002) http://www.childwise.co.uk. (215)

Barfe, L. (1998) *The under-16s market: 1998 Market Report.* Middlesex, Key Note Ltd, Hampton. (215)

Alissa Quart (2003) *Branded: The buying and selling of teenagers.* Arrow, London. (216)

Jill Matheson and Carol Summerfield (eds) (2000) *Social focus on young people.* National Statistics, London. (218, 226)

John Balding (2001) *Young People in 2001.* Schools Health Education Unit, Exeter. (218)

Mortimer, J.T. and Johnson, M.K. (1998) New perspectives on adolescent work and the transition to adulthood. In R. Jessor (ed) *New perspectives on adolescent risk behaviour.* Cambridge University Press, Cambridge. pp 425–498. (225)

Morrow, V. (1994) Responsible children: Aspects of Children's Work and Employment outside school in contemporary UK. In B. Mayall (ed) *Children's childhoods: Observed and experienced.* Falmer Press, London 128–143. (225)

David Coulter NSPCC (2002) *Personal Communication.* (227)

Michael Lewis (2001) *The Future Just Happened.* Hodder and Stoughton, London. (229)

Chapter 11

Future Foundation. *Report to reach for the sky.* August, 2002, Future Foundation, London. (231)

JUSTICE (1996) *Children and homicide.* Report of a Working Party. Justice, 59 Carter Lane, London, EC4V 5AQ. (236)

Matthews, H., Limb, M., Harrison, L., and Taylor, M. (1999) Local places and the political engagement of young people. *Youth and Policy,* **62**, 16–30. (238)

Carolyne Willow (1997) *Hear! Hear! Promoting Young People's Participation in Local Government.* Local Government Information Unit, London. (238)

Hugh Thomas (1977) Age and authority in Early Modern England. *Proceedings of the British Academy,* **LXII**, 205–48. (239)

Rachel Hodgkin and Peter Newell (1996) *Effective government structures for children.* Report of a Gulbenkian Foundation Inquiry. Calouste Gulbenkian Foundation, London. (239)

Michael Freeman (2001) *The child in family law.* In Julia Fionda (ed.) *Legal concepts of childhood.* Hart Publishing, Oxford. (241)

Virginia Morrow and Martin Richards (1996) *Transitions to adulthood: a family matter.* Joseph Rowntree Foundation, York. (251)

Telephone Helplines

General

Trust for the Study of Adolescence 01273 693311 (For general information, publications)

Parenting

National Family and Parenting Institute 0207 278 1920 (Information about parenting groups)

Young people in distress

ChildLine 0800 1111 (For children and young people in danger or distress).

Sexual health, contraception, pregnancy

Brook Advisory Service Helpline 0207 6178000 (For all sexual problems)

Drugs and alcohol

National Drugs HelpLine 0800 776600

ADFAM Helpline (Drugs) 0207 928 8900

Al Anon/Alateen Family Groups (Alcohol) 0207 403 0888
Accept (Alcohol) 0207 371 7477

Anorexia, bulimia
Eating Disorders Association 01603 765050

Mental health
Young Minds 0800 018 2138 (Information about mental health problems)

Advice on gay and lesbian issues
Lesbian and Gay Switchboard 0207 837 7324

Index